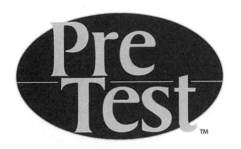

# Microbiology

PreTest™ Self-Assessment and Review

## Notice

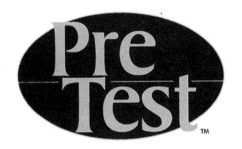

# Microbiology

## PreTest™ Self-Assessment and Review

### Twelfth Edition

**James D. Kettering, PhD**
Emeritus Professor
Loma Linda University
Loma Linda, CA

**Hansel M. Fletcher, PhD**
Professor of Microbiology and Associate Chairman—Microbiology
Department of Biochemistry and Microbiology
Loma Linda University
School of Medicine
Loma Linda, CA

**Craig A. Seheult, MS (Microbiology)**
Contributor—Immunology and Physiology/Molecular Microbiology
Loma Linda University
School of Medicine
Loma Linda, CA
Class of 2008

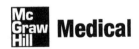 **Medical**

New York   Chicago   San Francisco   Lisbon   London   Madrid   Mexico City
Milan   New Delhi   San Juan   Seoul   Singapore   Sydney   Toronto

The *McGraw·Hill* Companies

**Microbiology: PreTest™ Self-Assessment and Review, Twelfth Edition**

1 2 3 4 5 6 7 8 9 0   DOC/DOC   0 9 8 7

ISBN-13: 978-0-07-147179-4
ISBN-10:    0-07-147179-0

*This book was set in Berkeley by International Typesetting and Composition.*
*The editors were Catherine A. Johnson and Regina Y. Brown.*
*The production supervisor was Sherri Souffrance.*
*Project management was provided by International Typesetting and Composition.*
*The cover designer was Maria Scharf.*
*Cover Photo: Bacteria © Cre8tive Studios / Alamy*
*RR Donnelley was printer and binder.*

*This book is printed on acid-free paper.*

**Library of Congress Cataloging-in-Publication Data**

Microbiology : PreTest self-assessment and review.—12th ed. / [edited by] James D. Kettering, Hansel M. Fletcher, Craig A. Seheult.
    p. ; cm.
Includes bibliographical references and index.
ISBN-13: 978-0-07-147179-4 (soft cover : alk. paper)
ISBN-10:    0-07-147179-0 (soft cover : alk. paper)
    1. Medical microbiology—Examinations, questions, etc.   2. Microbiology—Examinations, questions, etc.   3. Physicians—Licenses—Examinations—Study guides.
I. Kettering, James D.   II. Fletcher, Hansel M.   III. Seheult, Craig A.
    [DNLM: 1. Bacteria--Examination Questions.   2. Fungi--Examination Questions.
3. Parasites—Examination Questions.   4. Viruses—Examination Questions.
QW 18.2 M626      2007]
QR46.M544      2007
616.9'041076—dc22                                                                      2006033903

# Student Reviewers

**Grant E. Keeney**
University of Washington School of Medicine
Class of 2007

**Ranjith Ramasamy**
UMDNJ-Robert Wood Johnson Medical School
Class of 2007

**Farrant Sakaguchi**
University of Utah School of Medicine
Class of 2008

# Contents

# Immunology

# Introduction

Each *PreTest™ Self-Assessment and Review* allows medical students to comprehensively and conveniently assess and review their knowledge of a particular basic science, in this instance microbiology. The 500 questions parallel the format and degree of difficulty of the questions found in the United States Medical Licensing Examination (USMLE) Step 1. Practicing physicians who want to hone their skills before USMLE Step 3 or recertification may find this to be a good beginning in their review process. Each question is accompanied by an answer, a paragraph explanation, and a specific page reference to an appropriate textbook or journal article. A bibliography listing sources can be found following the last chapter of this text.

Each multiple-choice question in this book contains four or more possible answer options. In each case, select the ONE BEST ANSWER to the question.

An effective way to use this PreTest™ is to allow yourself one minute to answer each question in a given chapter. As you proceed, indicate your answer beside each question. By following this suggestion, you approximate the time limits imposed by the Step 1 exam.

After you finish going through the questions in the section, spend as much time as you need verifying your answers and carefully reading the explanations provided. Pay special attention to the explanations for the questions you answered incorrectly, but read every explanation. The authors of this material have designed the explanations to reinforce and supplement the information tested by the questions. If you feel you need further information about the material covered, consult and study the references indicated.

The High-Yield Facts added for this edition are provided to facilitate rapid review of microbiology. It is anticipated that the reader will use the High-Yield Facts as a "memory jog" before proceeding through the questions.

# Acknowledgments

The author wishes to thank Betty J. Kettering, MSPH, and David E. Kettering, J.D., for expert assistance in the production of the manuscript for this revision.

# High-Yield Facts

## PHYSIOLOGY AND MOLECULAR BIOLOGY

- Koch's postulates: (1) Specific organism must be in diseased animal; (2) organism must be isolated in pure culture; (3) organism produces disease in healthy susceptible animal; (4) organism reisolated from infected animal.
- Gram stain: (1) Fixation; (2) crystal violet; (3) iodine treatment; (4) decolorization (alcohol/acetone); (5) counterstain (safranin). Gram-positive = purple; gram-negative = red.
- Gram stain poor for: *Chlamydia, Mycoplasma, Rickettsia, Treponema, Mycobacterium* (use acid-fast stain), *Legionella* (use silver stain).
- Bacterial shapes: Bacilli (rod), cocci (spherical), spirilla (spiral).
- Bacterial aggregates: Diplococci (e.g., Neisseriae), Streptococci (chains), tetrads (fours), Staphylococci (clusters), Sarcinae (cubes).
- Flagella: Monotrichous—single polar flagellum; lophotrichous—cluster of flagella at pole; amphitrichous—flagella at both poles; peritrichous—flagella encircling the cell.
- Type VII pili = F or sex pili; important in bacterial conjugation.
- Conjugation—DNA transferred from one bacterium to another; transduction—viral transfer of DNA from one cell to another; transformation—cellular uptake of purified DNA.
- Peptidoglycan (murein or mucopeptide) layer: Unique to prokaryotes, consists of glycan polymers of sugar N-acetylglucosamine (NAG) and N-acetylmuramic acid (NAM), and cross-linked by a short peptide. Cross-linking enzymes are transpeptidases (targets for $\beta$-lactam antibiotics).
- Bacterial structures: Peptidoglycan (support); cell wall/membrane (antigenic); outer membrane (lipopolysaccharide [LPS]/endotoxin); plasma membrane (oxidative/transport enzymes); ribosome (protein synthesis); periplasmic space (hydrolytic enzymes and $\beta$-lactamases); capsule (antiphagocytic, polysaccharide except *Bacillus anthracis,* which is D-glutamate); pilus/fimbria (adherence, conjugation); flagellum (motility); spore (heat, chemical, dehydration resistance, consists of dipicolinic acid); plasmid (genes for toxins, enzymes, antibiotic resistance); glycocalyx (adherence, made of polysaccharide); inclusion bodies (no membrane; store glycogen, polyphosphate, poly-$\beta$-hydroxybutyric acid).

- Gram-positive: Teichoic acid unique.
- Gram-negative: LPS/endotoxin unique.
- LPS/endotoxin: Lipid A covalently linked to polysaccharide core and then unique "O antigen" polysaccharide repeat; illicits acute-phase protein response in vivo (release of TNF-$\alpha$, IL-1, IL-6) causing fever, and the like.
- Lysozyme: Breaks down glycan backbone bonds of peptidoglycan ($\beta$1-4 bonds between NAM and NAG).
- Spheroplast: Partial cell-wall lysozyme digestion.
- Protoplast: Complete cell-wall lysozyme digestion.
- Geometric growth: Cell number = $a(2^n)$, where $a$ is number of starting cells, $n$ equals number of generations.
- Bacterial growth curves (four phases): (1) Lag (no cellular division, cell size increase); (2) exponential (regular doubling time, essential nutrients decrease, toxins increase); (3) stationary (cell division rate = cell death rate); (4) death (cell energy stores depleted, exponential death to low population equilibrium).
- Bacteriostatic: Agent inhibits multiplication, growth resumes upon removal of agent.
- Bactericidal: Agent kills bacteria, irreversible.
- Sterile: Free from all forms of life.
- Disinfectant: Chemical kills bacteria but toxic to tissue.
- Septic: Pathogenic organism present in living tissue.
- Aseptic: Pathogenic organism not present in living tissue. (Virology—No bacterial agents present)
- Passive transport: No energy, movement down concentration gradient, no carrier molecule.
- Active transport: Requires energy, against concentration gradient.
- Fluoride ion (water, toothpaste, and the like): Inhibits several cellular bacterial enzymes, especially enolase.
- Bacterial pathogenesis: (1) Antiphagocytic (cell-wall proteins—protein A in *Staphylococcus aureus* and protein M in *Streptococcus pyogenes,* capsules, pili/fimbriae); (2) adherence factors (pili/fimbriae, lipoteichoic acid, glycocalyx, adhesion); (3) enzymes (coagulase, collagenase, fibrinolysin, hyaluronidase, lecithinase, mucinase); (4) toxins (exotoxins, endotoxins/LPS).
- Exotoxins: Polypeptide, highly fatal, toxoids as vaccines, mostly heat labile, secreted, both gram-negative and gram-positive.

- Endotoxins: LPS, low toxicity, no toxoids, no vaccines, heat stable, released on lysis, only gram-negative.
- Free radicals of oxygen (superoxides) kill anaerobic bacteria exposed to air. Superoxide dismutase is a potent bacterial antioxidant. The peroxidases in bacteria are protective.
- Obligate anaerobes: Lack catalase and/or superoxide dismutase and susceptible to oxidative damage, foul smelling, produce gas in tissue (e.g., *Actinomyces, Bacteroides,* and *Clostridium*).
- Superoxide dismutase catalyzes: $2O_2^- + 2H^+ \rightarrow H_2O_2 + O_2$
- Catalase catalyzes: $2H_2O_2 \rightarrow 2H_2O + O_2$
- Myeloperoxidase catalyzes: $Cl^- + H_2O_2 \rightarrow ClO^- + H_2O$
- NADPH oxidase catalyzes: $NADPH + 2O_2 \rightarrow 2O_2^- + H^+ NADP^+$
- Sites of action of antimicrobial agents include cell-wall synthesis, cell-membrane integrity, DNA replication, protein synthesis, DNA-dependent RNA polymerase, folic acid metabolism.

## VIROLOGY

Virus basics—terms: virion, capsid, capsomere, nucleocapsid
- All DNA viruses are double-stranded (ds), except Parvovirus.
- All DNA viruses have linear DNA, except papovaviruses and hepadnaviruses.
- All RNA viruses have single-stranded RNA (ssRNA), except reoviruses.
- Segmented RNA viruses include orthomyxoviruses and reoviruses.
- Positive sense RNA (same as mRNA) include picornaviruses, caliciviruses, flaviviruses, retroviruses, and coronaviruses. All other RNA viruses are negative sense (need viral RNA polymerase).
- Obligate intracellular parasites, using viral receptors to attach to host cell receptors.
- Growth cycle: Attachment, entry, eclipse, maturation, release.
- Viral disease patterns: Acute, chronic, latent (persistent).
- DNA viruses grow in the host nucleus (except poxviruses).
- RNA viruses grow in the host cytoplasm (except influenza and retroviruses).

### Hepatitis Viruses
- Hepatitis A (HAV)—RNA picornavirus, fecal-oral transmission, no chronic carriers.

- Hepatitis B (HBV)—DNA hepadnavirus, parental, sexual transmission passes through placenta, acute and chronic disease, HBV possesses a reverse transcriptase polymerase.
- Hepatitis C (HCV)—Flavivirus, +ssRNA, parental, sexual transmission, acute and chronic disease.
- Hepatitis D (HDV)—"Delta" hepatitis—defective RNA virus, requires HBV coinfection, acute and chronic infections.
- Hepatitis E (HEV)—Calicivirus, +ssRNA, fecal-oral transmission.

HAV and HBV have approved vaccines.

## DNA Viruses

- Parvovirus B19—ssDNA—causes fifth disease/erythema infectiosum (slapped cheek appearance).
- Papovaviruses.
  - Papillomaviruses—ds circular DNA—cause warts (human papillomavirus [HPV] type 1, 4—benign; 6, 11—anogenital; 16, 18—cervical carcinoma).
  - Polyoma viruses—BK—kidney disease; JC (progressive multifocal leukoencepalopathy).
- Adenovirus (ds linear DNA)—conjunctivitis and respiratory diseases in kids. Strains 10, 41 cause gastroenteritis.
- Herpesviruses.
  - Herpes simplex—latent infections common; "Shingles"—dermatomal distribution.
  - HSV-1—trigeminal ganglia; cold sores, conjunctivitis, and encephalitis (treat with acyclovir).
  - HSV-2—sacral nerve ganglia—sexually transmitted.
  - Varicella—zoster—chickenpox-shingles—lesions are asynchronous (all forms present). Vaccine attenuated.
  - Cytomegalovirus (CMV)—common; direct and sexual contact for transmission; retinitis and pneumonitis in immunocompromised; neonates—CMV inclusion disease.
  - Epstein-Barr virus (EBV)—infects B lymphocytes; causes infectious mononucleosis; positive for heterophile antibodies—EBV—early antigen (EA), viral capsid antigen (VCA), epstein barr nuclear antigen (EBNA)—diagnostic value.
- Poxviruses—largest, most complex virsus, dsDNA—grow in cytoplasm, complex envelope.

- Variola—smallpox, extinct since 1977. Bioterrorism agent. Vaccinia virus—vaccine strain.
- Molluscum contagiosum—benign tumors.

## Positive ssRNA Viruses
- Picornavirus (+ssRNA).
  - Polio, coxsackie A and B, echoviruses, HAV—polio—Salk/Sabin vaccines; the United States now uses killed vaccine.
  - All strains cause upper respiratory infections (URIs), rashes, limited central nervous system (CNS) infections (glucose normal; protein—elevated slightly); gastrointestinal (GI), hemorrhagic conjunctivitis, and myocarditis.
- Rhinoviruses—common cold.
  - Flaviviruses—HCV, yellow fever, dengue, Saint Louis encephalitis.
  - Togaviruses—Western Equine encephalitis, Eastern Equine encephalitis, Venezuelan Equine encephalitis, West Nile virus (birds and horses—normal hosts).
  - Rubella virus—German measles—(no insect vector)—causes severe birth defects.
  - Coronaviruses—common cold mostly; also severe acute respiratory syndrome (SARS).
  - Retroviruses—diploid genome—*gag* genes—p24, p7, p9, and p17; env—gp 120 and gp 41; *pol* gene reverse transcriptase/integrase; progene-protease AIDS (CD4) <200 lymphocytes/mm$^3$. Opportunistic infections—*Candida, Mycobacterium* species, multiple viruses, and protozoan.

## Negative ssRNA Viruses
- Require virion-associated RNA-dependent RNA polymerase.
- Paramyxoviruses.
  - Measles—fever, conjunctivitis, Koplic's spots—rash.
  - Complications—pneumonia, encephalitis; good vaccine.
  - Mumps—salivary, parotid glands; orchitis; good liver vaccine.
  - Respiratory syncytial virus—major cause of URI—infants (treat with ribovirin).
- Rhabdovirus—bullet-shaped—U.S. reservoirs—skunks, raccoons, foxes, coyotes/dogs, and bats; animal bite transmission; control animal vectors; Negri body—eosinophilic intracytoplasmic inclusion body.
- Orthomyxoviruses.
- Influenza A and B, segmented genomes.

- Genetic drift—minor antigen changes; genetic shift—major new hemagglutinin and/or neuraminidase changes.
- Bunyaviruses—California encephalitis virus; hantavirus.
- Arenaviruses—lymphocytic choriomenigitis virus, Lassa fever.

## dsRNA Viruses—Double-Shelled Capsids.

- Rotaviruses—infantile diarrhea.
- Reoviruses—common in humans, febrile diseases.

## BACTERIOLOGY

- Gram-positive cocci: Staphylococci catalase +, Streptococci catalase −.
- *S. aureus:* Mannitol-salt agar (selective and differential), yellow colonies, coagulase +, mannitol +, catalase +, some methicillin resistant, some vancomycin resistance emerging, protein A (binds IgG Fc inhibiting phagocytosis), rapid-onset food poisoning (enterotoxin), toxic shock syndrome, scalded skin syndrome, osteomyelitis, acute bacterial endocarditis (IV drug users), abscesses, recurrent infection in chronic granulomatous disease (CGD).
- *S. saprophyticus:* Second leading cause of urinary tract infection (UTI).
- Streptococci: β-hemolytic divided into groups (13 groups: A–O) based on cell-wall carbohydrate antigens. Group A divided into ≥50 types based on M proteins (virulence, specific immunity), catalase negative.
- *S. pyogenes* (group A): Hyaluronic acid capsule, carbohydrate antigen, M protein, bacitracin sensitive, cellulitis, rheumatic fever, glomerulonephritis, necrotizing fasciitis, erysipelas, scarlet fever.
- *Streptococcus viridans:* Normal oral flora, α-hemolytic, subacute bacterial endocarditis after dental/oral surgery.
- Enterococcus (*Streptococcus*) *faecalis* (group D): Normal intestinal flora, subacute bacterial endocarditis after pelvic/abdominal surgery, UTIs, growth in 6.5% NaCl.
- *Streptococcus agalactiae* (group B): Normal vaginal flora; in dairy products (cattle pathogen); neonatal sepsis; Christie, Atkins, Munch-Peterson (CAMP) test+.
- Peptostreptococci: Normal oral/vaginal flora, endocarditis, lung abscess.
- *Streptococcus pneumoniae:* Pneumonia, meningitis, otitis media (children), optochin sensitive, bile soluble, use quellung reaction, pneumococcal polyvalent vaccine.
- Dick test: Test susceptibility to scarlet fever.
- Shultz-Charlton test: Determine if rash is due to erythrogenic toxin of scarlet fever.

- Gram-negative cocci (*Neisseria*): Oxidase +, diplococci, polysaccharide capsule, associated with C5, 6, 7, 8 complement deficiency; pathogenic forms: Thayer-Martin agar −, chocolate agar +, nutrient agar −, 37°C growth +, room temperature −; nonpathogenic forms: Thayer-Martin agar −, chocolate agar +, nutrient agar +, 37°C growth +, room temperature +.
- *Neisseria meningitidis:* Capsule, endotoxin, toxemia, petechiae, hemorrhage, disseminated intravascular coagulation (DIC).
- Bacterial meningitis in <40-year-old = *S. pneumoniae;* >40-year-old = *S. pneumoniae;* 2–60 months = neonates = Group B streptococci, *E. coli;* neonates to 5-year-old young adults = *N. meningitidis.*
- *Neisseria gonorrhoeae:* Pili, IgA protease, pharyngitis, proctitis, pelvic inflammatory disease (PID), urethritis, cervicitis.
- Gram-positive Bacilli: Aerobic (Bacilli); anaerobic (*Clostridium*), killed by autoclave.
- *B. anthracis:* Polypeptide capsule, exotoxin, anthrax (wool-sorters' disease).
- *Bacillus cereus:* Food poisoning (food reheated once), enterotoxin.
- *Clostridium:* No cytochrome enzymes, no catalase, no superoxide dismutase.
- *Clostridium tetani:* Noninvasive, neurotoxins (prevents release of neural inhibitory transmitters such as γ-aminobutyric acid [GABA] and glycine), lockjaw, spastic paralysis, give toxoid/antitoxin.
- *Clostridium botulinum:* Noninvasive, exotoxins (prevents acetylcholine release), flaccid paralysis, antitoxin (honey ingestion).
- *Clostridium perfringens:* Invasive, enterotoxin, food poisoning, myonecrosis, collagenase, lecithinase, gas gangrene.
- *Clostridium difficile:* Pseudomembranous colitis, can occur after broad-spectrum antibiotic usage.
- *Corynebacterium diphtheria:* Gram-positive rod, metachromatic granules, exotoxin (inhibits EF-2 and protein synthesis).
- *Listeria monocytogenes:* Gram-positive rod in cerebrospinal fluid (CSF), compromised host, neonate, diarrhea after eating raw cheeses.
- *Salmonella:* Gram-negative rod, enteric fever, food poisoning; *Salmonella typhi* = human pathogen; other species = animal pathogens; motile; nonlactose fermenter.
- *Shigella:* Gram-negative rod, more virulent than *Salmonella*, bloody diarrhea, shigellosis is human disease, oral-anal route (fingers, flies, food, and feces), toxin inhibits protein synthesis.
- *E. coli:* Gram-negative rod, most common UTI, sepsis (serious); enterohemorrhagic *E. coli* (EHEC) (colitis, hemolytic uremic syndrome-verotoxin,

hamburger, beef); enteroinvasive *E. coli* (EIEC) (fever, bloody stool, diarrhea); enterotoxigenic *E. coli* (ETEC) (traveler's diarrhea); Enteropathogenic *E. coli* (EPEC) (infant fever and diarrhea, nonbloody stool).

- *Pseudomonas aeruginosa:* Gram-negative rod, antibiotic resistance, pigments, UTI, wounds, burns, greenish-yellow sputum.
- *Klebsiella:* Large capsule, UTI, pneumonia, especially in alcoholics.
- *Haemophilus influenzae:* Gram-negative rod, meningitis, otitis, sinusitis, epiglottitis.
- *Proteus:* Gram-negative rod, urease (urea → $NH_3$)—also produced by *Helicobacter pylori* and *Ureaplasma urealyticum;* UTI, wounds, renal stones.
- *Gardnerella vaginalis:* "Clue cells"; vaginitis with discharge (fishy smell).
- *Bordetella pertussis:* Capsule, pili, killed vaccine, whooping cough.
- *Yersinia pestis:* "Safety pin" (bipolar staining), plague (bubonic/pneumonic), rat flea.
- *Francisella tularensis:* Skinning rabbits (jackrabbits), tularemia.
- *Pasteurella multocida:* Cat/dog bites; cellulitis, "shipping fever."
- *Brucella:* Dye sensitivity test, undulant fever.
- *Mycobacterium tuberculosis:* Tuberculosis, acid-fast stain, Lowenstein-Jensen medium, purified protein derivative (PPD) testing.
- *Mycobacterium leprae:* Leprosy, cannot be cultured.
- *Haemophilus ducreyi:* Painful lesion, chancroid (syphilis: painless chancre).
- *Treponema pallidum:* Venereal Disease Research Laboratories (VDRL), Fluorescent Treponemal Antibody Absorption (FTA-ABS), IgM antibody, use penicillin G, three stages, spirochetes, dark-field microscopy.
- *Borrelia:* Aniline dyes (Wright's/Giemsa), *Ixodes* tick, relapsing fever, Lyme disease, acute necrotizing ulcerative gingivitis, spirochete.
- *Legionella pneumophila:* Legionnaires' disease, fulminating pneumonia, gram-negative rod, airborne through contaminated water (air-conditioner cooling system).
- Exotoxin: Heat labile.
- Endotoxin (LPS): Heat stable.
- Diphtheria/*Pseudomonas* exotoxin: Act via ADP-ribosylation of EF-2, thus protein synthesis inhibited.
- *E. coli, Vibrio cholerae, B. cereus* heat-labile enterotoxin: ADP-ribosylation of $G_s$ protein turns $G_s$ protein on, thus activating adenylate cyclase, leading to ↑cAMP and diarrhea.
- *B. pertussis* heat-labile enterotoxin: ADP-ribosylation of $G_i$ protein turns off $G_i$ protein, thereby activating adenylate cyclase, leading to ↑cAMP and diarrhea.

- *Vibrio:* Oxidase positive; one flagellum; curved, "comma-shaped" gram-negative rod; halophilic (except *V. cholerae*).
- *Vibrio parahaemolyticus:* Contaminated seafood, diarrhea.
- *Vibrio vulnificus:* Contaminated marine animals (oyster ingestion), diarrhea, skin lesions (handling).
- Vancomycin-resistant enterococci, methicillin-resistant *S. aureus* (MRSA), and vancomycin-indeterminate *S. aureus* (VISA) are among the most feared nosocomial pathogens. A recently introduced antibiotic, quinapristin-delfapristin, effectively treats vancomycin-resistant enterococci or the few vancomycin-indeterminate MRSAs that have occurred. Tx of MRSA is vancomycin.
- Following an upsurge of tuberculosis in the early 1990s, cases of *M. tuberculosis* infection have remained static. *M. tuberculosis* causes initial primary pulmonary infection as well as a chronic disease characterized by hemoptysis, loss of weight, and fever.
- Penicillin-resistant pneumococci (*S. pneumoniae*) may account for up to 40% of isolates of *S. pneumoniae*. Third- or fourth-generation cephalosporins may be used as alternative treatment as well as vancomycin and rifampin.
- *Campylobacter* and *Helicobacter* are both helical-shaped bacteria. *Helicobacter* is known to play a role in the pathogenesis of peptic ulcer disease, while *Campylobacter* causes a food-borne GI illness, most commonly from undercooked meat. Both bacteria are susceptible to antibiotics such as tetracycline. *Helicobacter* may be treated with Pepto-Bismol, metronidazole, and amoxicillin.

## RICKETTSIAE, CHLAMYDIAE, MYCOPLASMAS

### Rickettsiae

- *Rickettsia, Coxiella, Bartonella* (*Rochalimaea*), and *Ehrlichia*—main genera. All are obligate intracellular parasites due to limited ATP production. Insect vectors include ticks, mites, body lice.
- Rocky Mountain spotted fever—*Rickettsia rickettsii*—spread by ticks, invades capillaries, causing vasculitis. Rash commonly moves from extremities to trunk. Diagnosis is usually serology, using cross-reacting antibodies to *Proteus vulgaris* OX strains.
- Treat with tetracyclines.
- *Coxiella burnetii*—reservoir is livestock; inhalation transmission. Causes Q fever, an atypical pneumonia.

- *Bartonella*—pericellular, not intracellular infection. (*Bartonella quintana, Bartonella henselae*) Causes trench fever, septicemia, cat-scratch disease.
- *Ehrlichia*—infects monocytes, granulocytes; tick transmission.

## Chlamydiae

- Obligate intracellular parasites that do not produce ATP. Possess a modified gram-negative cell wall. A true bacterium.
- Unusual life cycle—infectious elementary bodies bind to receptors, enter cells, forming an intracellular reticulate body. Dividing reticulate bodies form new elementary bodies. Reticulate bodies form inclusion bodies in the host cell.
- *Chlamydia trachomatis*—Sensitive to sulfa drugs, stain with iodine (glycogen staining). Serotypes A, B, C cause trachoma, a chronic follicular keratoconjunctivitis, often resulting in blindness.
- Serotypes D–K cause reproductive tract infections, pneumonia, inclusion conjunctivitis. Chlamydial genital infections are widespread and common. Neonatal infections often result in inclusion conjunctivitis. Treat with erythromycins or tetracyclines.
- Serotypes L1, L2, and L3 cause lymphogranuloma venereum.
- Identify genital infections with molecular probes, fluorescent antibody (FA) staining for tissues, grow in McCoy cell cultures.
- *Chlamydia psittaci* uses birds as primary hosts. Humans develop an atypical pneumonia from inhaling the organism. Diagnosis is usually serology, not iodine staining.
- *Chlamydia pneumoniae* (TWAR)—human bronchitis, pneumonia, sinusitis. Treat with azithromycin.

## Mycoplasma

Bacteria with no cell wall.
- Grown on laboratory media; do not Gram stain.
- *Mycoplasma pneumoniae*—causes sore throat through atypical pneumonia (walking pneumonia). Treat with tetracyclines or erythromycins.
- *U. urealyticum*—urethritis, prostatitis. Tiny colonies.
- Free radicals of oxygen (superoxides) kill anaerobic bacteria exposed to air. Superoxide dismutase is a potent bacterial antioxidant. The peroxidases in bacteria are protective.
- Obligate anaerobes: Lack catalase and/or superoxide dismutase and susceptible to oxidative damage, foul smelling, produce gas in tissue (e.g., *Actinomyces, Bacteroides,* and *Clostridium*).

- Superoxide dismutase catalyzes: $2O_2^- + 2H^+ \rightarrow H_2O_2 + O_2$
- Catalase catalyzes: $2H_2O_2 \rightarrow 2H_2O + O_2$
- Myeloperoxidase catalyzes: $Cl^- + H_2O_2 \rightarrow ClO^- + H_2O$
- NADPH oxidase catalyzes: $NADPH + 2O_2 \rightarrow 2O_2^- \rightarrow H^+ NADP^+$
- Sites of action of antimicrobial agents include cell-wall synthesis, cell-membrane integrity, DNA replication, protein synthesis, DNA-dependent RNA polymerase, folic acid metabolism.

## MYCOLOGY

- Fungi (molds and yeasts) are eukaryotic—cell membranes have ergosterol (not cholesterol); target for imidazole, amphoteracin B, and nystatin antifungal.
- Fungal structures—hyphae (molds) or yeast.
  - Dimorphism—change from hyphae to yeast forms.
  - Hyphae grow into a mycelium; septate—cross-walls in hyphae; nonseptate—no cross-walls.
  - Yeasts—oval cells that replicate by budding.
  - Spores—reproductive devices—blastoconidia—yeast buds, conidia—hyphae, (macro- and microforms); endospores—*Coccidioides immitis;* arthroconidia—hyphae fragmentation.
- Laboratory—Sabouraud's agar-standard fungal medium.
  - Identity—based on morphology, biochemical test, immunologic tests, or genetic probes.
- Dermatophytes.
  - *Malassezia furfur*—hypopigmentation of skin.
  - *Trichophyton*—skin, hair, nails; *Microsporum*—hair and skin; *Epidermophyton*—nail and skin.
  - Tineas—ringworm (*Tinea capitis*—hair, Tinea corporis—skin, *Tinea cruris*—groin, *Tinea pedis*—foot).
  - *Candida*—pseudohyphae and yeast forms—normal flora—opportunist in immunocompromised patients.
  - *Sporothrix schenckii*—dimorphic fungus—plants—transmission on thorns, and the like, lymphotics involved.
- Thermally dimorphic fungi—systemic infections, rose gardeners disease.
  - *Histoplasma capsulatum*—fungus in the environment with tuberculate macroconidia; small, oval budding yeast in cells of the RES.
  - Central United States—river valleys, especially important—birds and caves.
    - Primary disease—asymptomatic to pneumonia.

- Systematic—especially in AIDS patients with mucocutaneous lesions common.
- Laboratory—history plus blood smears and culture.
- *C. immitis*—environment (southwest United States—sandy, deserts especially)—hyphae develop into arthroconidia; inhaled arthroconidia develop into spherules (endospores).
  - Primary disease—(valley fever)—asymptomatic to self-limited pneumonia; disseminated form (certain HLA types, pregnancy, and immunocompromised)—to skin, bone, joints, and meninges).
  - Laboratory—culture (hazardous); sputum, urine, bronchial washes may show spherules.
- *Blastomyces dermatitidis*—environment—hyphae with conidia on stalks; tissue—large yeast with broad-based bud.
  - Same geographical area as *Histoplasma conidia* are inhaled.
  - Primary disease—pneumonia.
  - Laboratory—large yeast, broad-based buds.

## Opportunistic Fungi
- *Aspergillus fumigatus*—hyphae with branches at acute angles and small conidia. Ubiquitous in environment. Fungus balls in lung cavities; invasive disease possible.
- *Candida albicans*—yeast and pseudohyphae normal mucocutaneous flora—oral thrush (infants and antibiotic users).
- Endocarditis—IV drug abusers/indwelling catheters.
- *Cryptococcus neoformans*—yeast with large capsule.
  - Environment—soil with bird droppings.
  - Disease—pulmonary (often asymptomatic) in pigeon breeders; fungal meningitis in AIDS patients and cancer patients.
  - Laboratory—latex agglutination—CSF (capsule antigen); india ink wet mount—capsules.
- *Mucor, Rhizopus, Absidia*—nonseptate hyphae.
  - Environment—common organisms.
  - Opportunists—rhinocerebral infections.
  - Laboratory—broad, nonseptate hyphae with 90° angles on branching.
- *Pneumocystis carinii*—exposure common—seldom disease except in immunocompromised (AIDS patients, and the like). Interstitial pneumonia presentation.
  - Laboratory—H and E tissue stains, silver stains, cup shaped cysts, Tx-TMP-SMX, pentamidine.

# PARASITOLOGY

- Protozoa are single-celled animals; trophozoites are motile, while cysts are involved in transmission.
- Amebas.
  - *Entamoeba histolytica*—disease of the large intestine; amebic dysentery—trophozoites feed on red blood cells (RBCs), causing ulcers. Also liver and lung abscesses possible.
  - *Naegleria*—free-living ameba in hot-water sources; primary amebic meningoencephalitis (PAM). Rapid onset of symptoms, with death possible in days.
  - Acanthamoeba—free-living amebas.
- Flagellates.
  - *Giardia lamblia*—worldwide distribution, animal reservoirs. Cysts in water sources; trophozoites attach to intestine, causing watery diarrhea and malabsorption. Cramping, light-colored, fatty stools. Also in day-care centers.
  - *Trichomonas vaginalis*—Trophozoite with undulating membrane and polar flagella. Presents with fishy-smelling, yellow discharge. Males usually asymptomatic, sexually transmitted.
  - *Trypanosoma*—flagellates, tsetse fly vector. African sleeping sickness.
  - *Trypanosoma cruzi*—Chagas' disease, kissing bug vector. South and Central America, cardiomegaly.
  - *Leishmania*—sandfly vectors. Visceral, cutaneous, and mucocutaneous lesions.
- Sporozoans—sexual and asexual life cycle forms.
  - *Cryptosporidium parvum*—U.S. waters, causes a self-limited diarrhea.
  - *Plasmodium* species cause malaria. *Anopheles* mosquito vectors. Complicated life cycles. *Plasmodium vivax, Plasmodium ovale, Plasmodium malariae, Plasmodium falciparum*.
  - *Toxoplasma gondii*—reservoir is cats. Humans ingest cysts from cat feces or undercooked meats. Special danger in human fetus congenital development.
- Flukes.
  - *Fasciolopsis buski*—intestinal, cysts on water plants ingested, diarrhea.
  - *Clonorchis sinensis*—liver, from raw or undercooked fish. Biliary tree localization and liver location.
  - *Fasciola hepatica*—sheep liver fluke. Ingestion of metacercariae on aquatic plants.
  - *Schistosoma*—blood flukes, *Schistosoma hematobium* cystitis.

- Cestodes—segmented flatworms with complicated life cycles.
  - *Taenia solium* (pork) and *Taenia saganata* (beef)—larval forms in undercooked meat. Adult tapeworms develop in the intestine.
  - *Diphyllobothrium latum*—fish tapeworm. Fish in freshwater lakes, undercooked fish ingested. Depletes host of vitamin $B_{12}$.
  - *Echinococcus granulosis*—tissue cestode. Humans are intermediate hosts and ingest eggs from sheepdog feces, hydatid cysts of liver.
- Nematodes—roundworms.
  - *Ascaris lumbricoides*—may cause intestinal blockage.
  - *Enterobius vermicularis* (pinworm)—eggs in bedclothing, etc. Autoinoculation common. Widespread in the United States.
  - *Necator americanus*—New World hookworm.
  - *Ancylostoma duodenale*—Old World hookworm. Eggs in soil, penetrate bare feet.
  - *Strongyloides stercoralis* (threadworm)—tropics, southwest United States, similar to hookworms, no eggs, only larval forms.
  - *Trichuris trichiura* (whipworm)—tropics. Eggs ingested, poor sanitation. Causes mucoid or bloody diarrhea.
  - *Trichinella spiralis* (pork roundworm)—larvae ingested in pork or wild game meat. Larvae may calcify in muscle of intermediate host.
- Tissue nematodes—filarial worms. None are significant in the United States.
  - *Onchocerca volvulus*—river blindness, blackfly vector, Treatment-Ivermectin.
  - *Loa loa*—biting fly vector.
  - *Wuchereria bancrofti*—mosquito vectors. May cause elephantiasis.

## IMMUNOLOGY

- Two types of immune response: (1) Adaptive or acquired (specific), (2) innate (native or nonadaptive).
- Innate immunity: Nonspecific, no immunological memory, first line of defense (epithelial), biochemical defenses (stomach ↓pH, GI proteolytic enzymes, and bile), phagocytes (polymorphonuclear neutrophils [PMNs] and monocytes, macrophages), Soluble mediators (complement, acute-phase proteins such as C-reactive protein, cytokines such as ILs, IFNs, CSFs), inflammation (C5a: chemotaxis, C3b: opsonization, neutrophils.
- Adaptive immunity: Specific, antigen-driven, possesses discrimination and memory, divided into (1) humoral immunity (B cells, plasma cells) and (2) cell-mediated immunity (T helper, T cytotoxic).

- Antibodies (B lymphocytes/plasma cells): Main functions are (1) *neutralize* toxins/viruses, (2) *opsonize* bacteria, (3) *complement activation.*
- Antibodies (five isotypes): IgG, IgA, IgM, IgD, IgE (based on Fc heavy-chain differences), two light chains and two heavy chains held together by S-H bridges, hinge region is polyproline, paratope binds antigen and is composed of heavy and light chain. Pepsin yields $F(ab)_2$, papain yields two "useless arms."
- Antibody concentrations (serum): IgG > IgA > IgM > IgD > IgE.
- IgG: Transplacental (Rh incompatibility, hemolytic disease of newborn), 80% of serum antibody, binds (activates) complement, four subclasses, main antibody in secondary response.
- IgA: Secretory antibody, serum (monomer), secretions (dimers), two subclasses, dimer (J chain), does not bind complement.
- IgM: Pentamer, binds complement, first to appear after infection, elevated in congenital/perinatal infections.
- IgD: Susceptible to proteolytic degradation, found with surface IgM on mature B lymphocytes.
- IgE: Cytotropic/reaginic antibody, allergy antibody, type I hypersensitivity (mast cells/basophils protective in worm infections), lowest concentration in serum.
- Bence Jones proteins: Multiple myeloma—large amounts of $\kappa/\gamma$ light chains in urine excretion.
- Natural killer cells: Marker is CD16 (IgG Fc receptor).
- B cells: Antibody producers contributing to allergy (IgE), autoimmunity, host defense (opsonize, neutralize, complement activate).
- B cell markers: Fc receptor, C3 receptor, CD21 (receptor for EB virus), CD10 (common acute lymphoblastic leukemia antigen (CALLA).
- T cells: Host defense (fungi, viruses, *M. tuberculosis*), allergy (type IV), antibody regulation, graft/tumor rejection.
- T cell markers: CD2, TCR$\alpha\beta$-CD3, CD4 (HIV) or CD8, CD44 (migration).
- Complement deficiencies: (1) C1 esterase inhibitor: angioedema; (2) decay-accelerating factor (DAF): paroxysmal nocturnal hemoglubinuria; (3) C3: severe, recurrent infections (sinus and respiratory)-pneumonococce; (4) C5-9: disseminated gonococcemia.
- Major histocompatibility complex (MHC) Class I: Exists on all nucleated cells.
- MHC Class II: Exists on antigen-presenting cells (macrophages/dendritic cells), important to organ rejection.

- Cytokines: IFN (antiviral), TNF (inflammation, fever, acute-phase reactants, cachexia), IL-1 (fever/pyrogen, acute-phase proteins), IL-2 (T cell stimulator), IL-3 (bone marrow stimulator), IL-4 (IgE production), IL-5 (proeosinophil, antihelminths), IL-6 (acute-phase proteins, B cell differentiation), IL-8 (inflammation, chemotaxis), IL-12 (NK cell stimulator, $T_H1$ stimulator, active cytotoxic lymphocyte stimulator, promotes cell-mediated immunity).
- Acute-phase cytokines: IL-1, IL-6, TNF-$\alpha$.
- Mitogens: B lymphocytes (LPS), T lymphocytes (phytohemagglutinin [PHA] and Con A), both B and T cells (pokeweed mitogen [PWM]).
- Enzyme-linked immunosorbent assay (ELISA) presumptive diagnosis of HIV infection, Western blot definitive diagnosis of HIV infection → both detecting anti-HIV antibodies in patient sera; detection of HIV RNA by nucleic acid amplification of viral load is best predictor of "progression to AIDS."
- Immunodeficiencies: (1) Primary—rare and *cause* disease; (2) secondary—common and the *result* of disease.
- Primary immunodeficiencies: Bruton's agammaglobulinemia—no B cells, low antibodies, small tonsils, only males; DiGeorge's syndrome (congenital thymic aplasia)—third and fourth pharyngeal pouches development failure, no thymus, no T cells, no parathyroid (hypocalcemia), and recurrent viral, fungal, protozoal infections; severe combined immunodeficiency disease (SCID)—no T or B cells, defective IL-2 receptor, deficiency adenosine enzyme, recurrent infections (viral, bacterial, fungal, protozoal); Wiskott Aldrich—B and T cell deficiency, low IgM, high IgA, normal IgE; ataxia telangiectasia—defective DNA repair; Chédiak-Higashi disease—autosomal-recessive defect in phagocytosis; CGD—NADPH oxidase deficiency, increased opportunistic pathogens, phagocytic deficiency; chronic mucocutaneous candidiasis—*C. albicans* T cell dysfunction.
- Immunodeficiency characterized by unusual and recurrent infections:
  - B cell (antibody) deficiency—bacterial infections.
  - T cell deficiency—viral, fungal, and protozoal infections.
  - Phagocytic cells deficiency—pyogenic infections (bacterial), skin infections, systemic bacterial opportunistic infections.
  - Complement deficiencies—pyogenic infections (bacterial).
- Hypersensitivity: (1) Type I (anaphylaxis, immediate-type hypersensitivity); (2) type II (cytotoxic hypersensitivity); (3) type III (immune complex hypersensitivity); (4) type IV (cell-mediated, delayed-type hypersensitivity).

- Type I: Mast cell/basophil, IgE, vasoactive amines, asthma, anaphylaxis, local wheal, and flare.
- Type II: IgM, IgG bind antigen and lyse cell, autoimmune hemolytic anemia, Goodpasture's syndrome, erythroblastosis fetalis.
- Type III: Immune complex, serum sickness, Arthus reaction → antibody-antigen complexes.
- Type IV: Lymphokines released from activated T lymphocytes, TB skin test, contact dermatitis, transplant rejection.
- Autoantibodies: Systemic lupus (antinuclear antibodies, anti-dsDNA, anti-Smith); drug-induced lupus (antihistone); rheumatoid arthritis (anti-IgG); celiac disease (antigliadin), Goodpasture's syndrome (antibasement membrane); Hashimoto's thyroiditis (antimicrosomal); scleroderma Calcinosis Raynaud Esophagus Sclerosis Teleangiectasiae (CREST) (anticentromere); scleroderma diffuse (anti-scl-70).
- Active immunity: Induced after exposure to foreign antigens, memory established, slow onset.
- Vaccines: (1) Capsular polysaccharide vaccines (*Streptococcus, N. meningitidis, H. influenzae*); (2) toxoid vaccines (*C. diphtheriae, C. tetani, B. pertussis*); (3) purified protein vaccines (*B. pertussis, Borrelia burgdorferi, B. anthracis*); (4) live, attenuated bacterial vaccines (*Mycobacterium bovis* for tuberculosis/BCG, *F. tularensis*); (5) killed bacterial vaccines (*V. cholerae, Y. pestis, R. rickettsiae*/typhus, *C. burnetii*/Q fever); (6) killed, live, attenuated, and polysaccharide vaccines (*S. typhi*).
- Adjuvants (human vaccines): Aluminum hydroxide or lipid.
- Passive immunity: Administration of preformed antibody in immune globulin preparations, no memory established, rapid onset (e.g., tetanus antitoxin, botulinum antitoxin, diphtheria antitoxin), antitoxin = immune globulins.

# Physiology and Molecular Microbiology

## Questions

**DIRECTIONS:** Each question below contains four or more suggested responses. Select the **one best** response to each question.

**1.** A 28 year-old female with folliculitis was not responsive to a 10-day treatment course with penicillin. Which of the following numbered bonds of the 6-amino-penicillanic acid (shown below) would be broken by the penicillinase isolated from the etiologic agent?

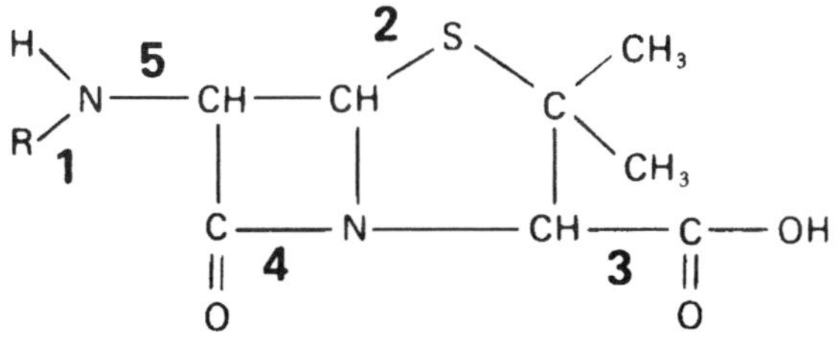

a. 1
b. 2
c. 3
d. 4
e. 5

**2.** Following an ineffective antibiotic therapy using glycopeptides, a gram-negative rod was isolated from a 35-year-old male who presented with symptoms of urinary tract infection. Which of the following bacterial transport methods is energy-independent and is most likely uninvolved in transport of the antibiotics into the cell?

a. ATP-dependent active transport
b. Facilitated diffusion
c. Group translocation
d. Proton gradient energized active transport
e. Simple diffusion

**3.** A 36-year-old male develops a painful purulent urethral discharge following a 2-week vacation to Thailand. A Gram stain reveals gram-negative diplococci. Iron is essential for the expression of its virulence factors. Which of the following macromolecules is important in iron metabolism?

a. Ferric oxide
b. Lactoferrin
c. Lipopolysaccharide (LPS)
d. Siderophores
e. Transferrin

**4.** A medical student is admitted to the emergency department with symptoms of hemorrhagic colitis. An aliquot of *Escherichia coli* strain, which is considered the etiologic agent of the infection, is treated with ethylenediaminetetraacetic acid (EDTA). The first wash is analyzed and found to contain alkaline phosphatase, DNase, and penicillinase. Which of the following is the anatomic area of the cell most likely affected by the EDTA?

a. Chromosome
b. Mesosomal space
c. Periplasmic space
d. Plasma membrane
e. Slime layer

## Item 5–7

A 52-year-old male develops abscess following surgery to repair an abdominal gunshot wound. Gram stain of the exudates from his foul-smelling abscess reveals numerous polymorphonuclear neutrophils (PMNs) and several gram-negative rods that did not grow on blood plates in the presence of $O_2$. Metabolism of $O_2$ results in toxic reactive oxygen species.

**5.** Which of the following enzymes is most likely involved in the following reaction?

$$2O^{2-} + 2H^+ \rightarrow H_2O_2 + O_2$$

a.  ATPase
b.  Catalase
c.  Oxygen permease
d.  Peroxidase
e.  Superoxide dismutase

**6.** Which of the following enzymes is most likely involved in the following reaction?

$$H_2O_2 + H_2A^* \rightarrow 2H_2O + A \text{ (“A” may be a number of chemical groups).}$$

a.  ATPase
b.  Flavoprotein oxidase
c.  Oxygen permease
d.  Peroxidase
e.  Superoxide dismutase

**7.** One of the bacteria isolated from the foul-smelling exudates taken from an abscess is missing superoxide dismutase, catalase, and a peroxidase. Which of the following statements best describes this microorganism?

a.  Aminoglycoside antibiotics will be effective against this bacterium
b.  This bacterium is a facultative aerobe
c.  This bacterium is an anaerobe
d.  This bacterium is more virulent than one containing the three enzymes
e.  This bacterium will survive in an $O_2$ environment

## Questions 8–9

A 20-year-old pregnant female patient presents to the emergency room with a 4-day history of fever, chills, and myalgia. Two days prior to this she had noted painful genital lesions. Pelvic examination revealed extensive vesicular and ulcerative lesions on the left labia minora and majora with marked edema. The cervix had exophytic (outward-growing) necrotic ulcerations. Specimens were taken to test for *Neisseria gonorrhoeae, Treponema pallidum, Haemophilus ducreyi, Chlamydia trachomatis,* and herpes simplex virus type 2 (HSV-2).

**8.** You decide to use newly purchased cutting-edge technology to rapidly identify the infecting pathogen. Real-time polymerase chain reaction requires which of the following reaction ingredient sets?

a.  Specimen (template DNA), forward primer, reverse primer, polymerase (Taq), dNTPs, $MgCl_2$ hepes buffer, $H_2O$, and fluorescent reporter (i.e., SYBR-green I)
b.  Specimen (template DNA), forward primer, reverse primer, polymerase (Taq), dNTPs, $MgCl_2$, hepes buffer, and $H_2O$
c.  Specimen (template DNA), forward primer only, polymerase (Taq), dNTPs, $MgCl_2$, hepes buffer, and $H_2O$
d.  Specimen (template DNA), reverse primer only, polymerase (Taq), dNTPs, $MgCl_2$, hepes buffer, and $H_2O$
e.  Specimen (template DNA), forward primer, reverse primer, dNTPs, $MgCl_2$, hepes buffer, $H_2O$, and fluorescent reporter (i.e., SYBR-green I)

**9.** Real-time SYBR-green polymerase chain reaction (PCR) reveals the following results:

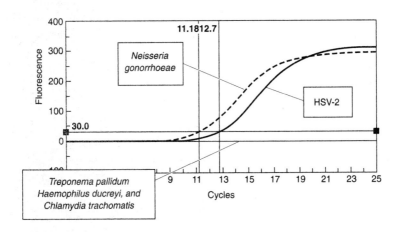

Which of the following is true?

a. The woman is infected with N. gonorrhoeae, T. pallidum, H. ducreyi, C. trachomatis, and herpes simplex virus type 2
b. The woman is infected with only HSV-2
c. The woman is infected with only N. gonorrhoeae
d. The woman is infected with both N. gonorrhoeae and herpes simplex type 2
e. The woman is not infected with any of the above-mentioned pathogens

**10.** A gram-negative diplococci identified as N. gonorrhoeae is isolated from an 18-year-old male who presented with symptoms of urethritis. Continuous passage of this strain on laboratory medium results in the reversion of a fimbriated to a nonfrimbriated strain. Which of the following is the most likely implication of this phenomena?

a. A negative capsule strain
b. Death of the organism
c. Inability of N. gonorrhoeae to colonize the mucosal epithelium
d. Loss of serologic specificity
e. Reversion to a gram-positive stain

**11.** Eighteen hours after eating undercooked chicken, a 50-year-old farmer presents to the emergency room with abdominal pain, cramping, bloody diarrhea, and nausea. An isolate from the stool is serologically recognized as *Salmonella enteritidis* serovar *newport*. A mutant of this organism has lost region 1 (O-specific polysaccharide) of its LPS. This mutant would be identified as which of the following?

a. *Arizona*
b. *Salmonella typhi*
c. *Salmonella newport*
d. *S. enteritidis*
e. *S. enteritidis* serovar *newport*

**12.** A 10-week-old infant is diagnosed with meningitis. A lumbar puncture reveals numerous neutrophils and gram-positive rods. She is admitted to the hospital and started on IV β-lactams. Which of the following targets would most likely play a role in the development of resistance to the antibiotics?

a. Bactoprenol
b. DNA gyrase
c. Penicillin-binding proteins (PBPs)
d. Reverse transcriptase
e. RNA polymerase

**13.** A cattle farmer develops necrotic lesions on his hands following a traumatic encounter with a bull. Selective inhibition of synthesis of dipicolinic acid (structure shown below) from the etieologic agent of the infection would most likely inhibit the formation of which of the following structures?

$$HOOC - \underset{N}{\bigcirc} - COOH$$

a. Bacterial flagella
b. Bacterial spores
c. Eukaryotic cilia
d. Eukaryotic flagella
e. Fimbriae

## Item 14–16

A 30-year-old male presents to the emergency room with high fever and malaise which he reports began 4 days ago and got progressively worse each day. He appears underweight and very ill. Physical examination reveals needle marks in both antecubial fossae. Listening for heart sounds, you hear a distinctive systolic heart murmur. You order blood cultures and make a presumptive diagnosis of acute bacterial endocarditis. Following is the growth curve of the organism growing in a nutrient medium at 35°C with both $O_2$ and added $CO_2$ present.

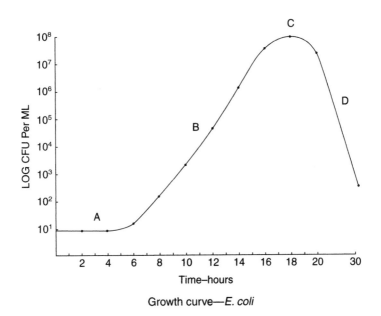

Growth curve—*E. coli*

The following descriptions are given for the phases of this bacterial growth curve:

A. Lag phase
B. Log phase
C. Stationary phase
D. Death phase

**14.** Which of the following phases would most likely be missing detectable growth and hence would be resistant to β-lactam antibiotics?

a. Lag phase
b. Log phase
c. Stationary phase
d. Death phase

**15.** On which of the following growth phases would treatment with gentamicin have a maximal effect?

a. Lag phase
b. Log phase
c. Stationary phase
d. Death phase

**16.** An outbreak of diarrhea is thought to be related to a group of vendors who were selling hotdogs at the county fair. Stool cultures are positive for *Salmonella* in almost all the patients. Growth of the isolated colonies in nutrient liquid medium without the transfer to fresh medium will eventally induce the death growth phase of the organism. Which of the following is a limiting factor in microbial growth?

a. Accumulation of oxygen-free radicals
b. Accumulation of peroxide
c. Accumulation of toxic products in the growth medium
d. Loss of superoxide dismutase
e. Oxygen

**17.** The successful treatment of infectious diseases is based on the principle of selective toxicity. Which of the following antimicrobial agents is the most toxic to humans?

a. Bacitracin
b. Cephalosporin
c. Mitomycin
d. Penicillin
e. Vancomycin

**18.** A 42-year-old alcoholic man presents with fever, chills, cough, and chest x-ray suggestive of pneumonia. The Gram-stained smear of sputum shows many PMNs and gram-positive cocci in pairs and chains. Which of the following is the correct order of the procedural steps when performing the Gram stain?

a.  Fixation, crystal violet, alcohol/acetone decolorization, safranin
b.  Fixation, crystal violet, iodine treatment, alcohol/acetone decolorization, safranin
c.  Fixation, crystal violet, iodine treatment, safranin
d.  Fixation, crystal violet, safranin
e.  Fixation, safranin, iodine treatment, alcohol/acetone decolorization, crystal violet

**19.** A 78-year-old man presents to the local emergency department with a severe headache and stiff neck. The CSF specimen is cloudy. Analysis reveals 400 white blood cells per cubic millimeter (95% PMNs), a protein concentration of 75 mg/dL, and a glucose concentration of 20 mg/dL. While in the ER, a resident does a Gram stain of the CSF but mistakenly forgets the iodine treatment step. If the meningitis is caused by *Streptococcus pneumoniae*, how will the bacteria seen on the resident's slide appear?

a.  All the cells will be blue
b.  All the cells will be decolorized
c.  All the cells will be purple
d.  All the cells will be red
e.  All the cells will lyse, thus no Gram stain results will be obtained
f.  Half of the cells will be red and the other half will be blue

**20.** A 28-year-old female just returned from a 1-week cruise with stops along the coast of Mexico. Forty-eight hours after her return she is reported to have headache, fever, abdominal cramps, and constipation. Over the next 5 days her fever increases with continued complaints of myalgias, malaise, and anorexia. A blood culture is positive for *S. typhi*. Her condition improves with a treatment course of a cephalosporin. Which of the following is the function of porins that would prevent the effective use of other antimicrobials ?

a.  Hydrolysis of hydrophilic antimicrobials
b.  Metabolism of phosphorylated intermediates
c.  Serologic stabilization of the O antigen
d.  Inactivation of hydrophobic antimicrobials
e.  Transfer of small molecules through the outer membrane

**21.** A 21-year-old man was bitten by a tick in Oregon. Two years later, during the course of routine screening for an unknown ailment, a screening Lyme disease test was performed, which was negative. A Western blot strip (IgG) showed the following pattern:

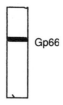

Gp66

Which of the following is the correct interpretation of the test?
a. The patient has acute Lyme disease
b. The patient has chronic Lyme disease
c. The patient should be tested for HIV on the basis of the Western blot
d. The pattern may represent nonspecific reactivity
e. The screening test should be repeated

**22.** Over 30 individuals attending a home improvement conference are hospitalized with bloody diarrhea and severe hematological abnormalities. An investigation establishes that all of these individuals developed symptoms following consumption of hamburgers from the same fast-food restaurant chain. Although other individuals ate the same hamburgers they did not report any symptoms. An analysis is initiated using PCR to evaluate the *E. coli* strains from all the individuals, looking for the major virulence factor associated with *E. coli* 0157/H7, the etiologic bacterium responsible for the outbreak. Early attempts at the PCR used *E. coli* DNA polymerase. This was replaced with DNA polymerase from *Thermus aquaticus* ("Taq" polymerase). Which of the following is the primary advantage in using this enzyme?
a. It is cheaper than *E. coli* polymerase
b. Specificity is increased because nonspecific hybridization of primers does not occur
c. Use of Taq polymerase enables lower temperatures to be used
d. Use of Taq polymerase results in fewer PCR cycles
e. Upon repeated cycling, Taq polymerase becomes denatured, which causes less interference with the hybridization process

### Item 23–25

A healthy 45-year-old female had root canal treatment about 3 weeks ago. She now presents with a new heart murmur, fever, painful skin nodules, and abdominal pain with abnormal liver function test. In addition, there are other systemic complications that cannot be attributed to α-hemolytic streptococci, the major suspected organism. Because several patients from the same county had a similar clinical presentation, an exploration for defining all the micoorganisms in the oral cavity is initiated.

You have been asked to design a nucleic acid amplification test for a rarely isolated bacterium. There are several questions that you must ask in order to develop a test that can be used to diagnose disease.

**23.** Assume, initially, that the PCR will amplify any DNA, human or microbial. Which of the following is the best way to prevent contamination of the PCR process?

a. Do all of the work under a hood
b. Incorporate self-sterilizing agents into the PCR mixture
c. Use universal precautions
d. Wash benches with bleach
e. Wear gloves

**24.** You must choose primers for this PCR. *Primers* are small pieces of nucleic acid that recognize a pair of unique sites on the bacterial chromosome. For an optimum test to be developed, which of the following characteristics is the least desirable?

a. Ability to be constructed by a synthesizer
b. Ability to serve as a template for replication
c. Complementary to sequences on the bacterial chromosome
d. That the sequences are widely recognized by many bacterial species
e. Uniqueness to the organism that you wish to detect

**25.** You have chosen the primers for the PCR that you designed. You have also developed a reaction mixture that contains, among other substances, a polymerase enzyme. After the primer pairs have been amplified, they must be detected. Which of the following detection methods is most sensitive (that is, will detect the highest number of amplicons)?

a. Capture of the amplicons on a solid phase followed by an enzyme immunoassay
b. Ethidium staining of the amplified products (amplicons)
c. Labeling of the amplicons with fluorescent dyes
d. Microscopy
e. Southern blot

**26.** *E. coli* is isolated from a urinary tract infection in a high school-aged young woman. Which one of the following statements about the *E. coli* cells shown in the photomicrograph below is true?

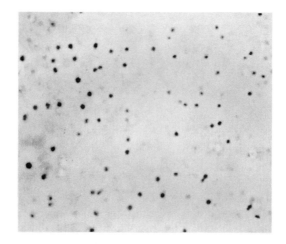

a. They are commonly referred to as endospores
b. They are osmotically stable
c. They can result from treatment with penicillin
d. They have formed cell walls but have become coccoid
e. Treatment of the parent *E. coli* with lysozyme has no effect

**27.** A 3-year-old girl from a family that does not believe in immunization presents to the emergency room with a sore throat, fever, malaise, and difficulty breathing. A gray membrane covering the pharynx is observed on physical examination. *Corynebacterium diphtheriae* is confirmed as the etiologic agent of this infection.

Analysis of the gene for the major virulence factor is needed by a graduate student for further study. The sequence of the cloning process is critical to the production of clones which will facilitate amplification of the cloned fragment. Which of the following steps initializes the cloning process?

a. Amplification of source DNA
b. Detection and purification of clones
c. Incorporation of a cloning vector into the host cell
d. Isolation and fragmentation/amplication of source DNA
e. Joining of host DNA to a cloning vector

**28.** A 3-year-old girl from a daycare center is brought to the local public health clinic because of a severe, intractable cough. During the previous 10 days, she had a persistent cold that had worsened. The cough developed the previous day and was so severe that vomiting frequently followed it. The child appears exhausted from the coughing episodes. A blood cell count shows a marked leukocytosis with a predominance of lymphocytes. To rule out the infection of other children and staff at the daycare, samples taken from them are evaluated with a *Bordetella* specific DNA probe. Which one of the following statements is usually true of nucleic acid probes?

a. Nucleic acid probes are not as sensitive as traditional culture methods for detection of pathogenic microorganisms
b. Only DNA can be used as a probe
c. Primers are labeled to allow detection, but probes are unlabeled
d. Probes can be designed so that they can detect very specific pieces of a nucleic acid, for example, a penicillin-resistant gene

**29.** A 55-year-old male presents with severe bilateral pulmonary infiltrate, elevated temperature leucocytosis, elevated enzymes, elevated creatine kinase. He and six of his friends had recently visited their favorite resturant, which had a large water fountain that was misty on the day of his visit. He is diagnosed with Legionnaires' disease; however, his friends do not yet have similar symptoms. To evaluate their infectious state, specimens are taken from these individuals and analysed by PCR. Which of the following is usually required for PCR?

a. A heat-sensitive DNA polymerase enzyme
b. A single nucleotide primer
c. An ultracentrifuge
d. A universal probe to detect the amplified product
e. Knowledge of the genetic sequence to be amplified

### Item 30–33

The following five growth curves are lettered (A–E) corresponding to an expected growth curve if certain antibiotics were added to an exponentially growing culture of *E. coli*. The arrow indicates when antibiotics were added to the growing culture.

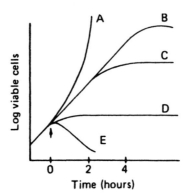

**30.** Chloramphenicol treatment would be expected to produce which one of the following growth curves?

a. A
b. B
c. C
d. D
e. E

**31.** Penicillin would be expected to produce which one of the following growth curves?

a. A
b. B
c. C
d. D
e. E

**32.** Sulfonamide would be expected to produce which one of the following growth curves?

a. A
b. B
c. C
d. D
e. E

**33.** If no antibiotics were added to the exponentially growing culture, which one of the following growth curves would result?

a. A
b. B
c. C
d. D
e. E

**34.** Several strains of *S. pneumoniae* are isolated from various patients. Some demonstrate high virulence while others appear to be nonvirulent. Mixing these cultures in the laboratory causes the nonvirulent strains to become pathogenic in laboratory animal experiments. Uptake by a recipient cell of soluble DNA released from a donor cell is defined as which of the following?

a. Competence
b. Conjugation
c. Recombination
d. Transduction
e. Transformation

**35.** A diphtheroid gram-positive rod may develop into a pathogenic *C. diphtheriae* by means of a bacteriophage infection. Transfer of a donor chromosome fragment by a temperate bacterial virus is defined as which one of the following?

a. Competence
b. Conjugation
c. Recombination
d. Transduction
e. Transformation

**36.** An increase in antibiotic resistance has been observed in microbial strains isolated from patients in medical centers. Direct transfer of a plasmid between two bacteria is defined as which of the following?

a. Competence
b. Conjugation
c. Recombination
d. Transduction
e. Transformation

**37.** After incubating a culture of five *E. coli* bacteria for 2 hours, the following graph was constructed. Which of the following represents the number of *E. coli* now present in this culture?

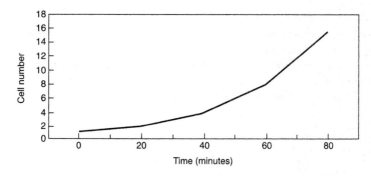

a. 32
b. 64
c. 160
d. 320
e. 640

**38.** Which of the following is true of Koch's postulates?

a. The causal organism must be isolated, grown in pure culture, cause disease in a healthy susceptible animal, and ultimately be recovered from the inoculated animal
b. The causal organism must be isolated, grown in pure culture, cause disease in a previously immunized (to the causal organism) animal, and ultimately be recovered from the inoculated animal
c. The causal organism need only be isolated and grown in pure culture
d. The causal organism may be inferred through an extensive history and physical of the diseased animal
e. The causal organism must cause repeated symptoms (illness) in the same (original) animal

**39.** The following diagram illustrates the cell wall of gram-negative bacteria.

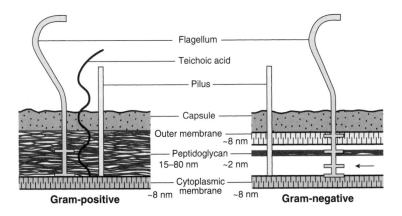

Which of the following statements is indicative of the contents of the indicated (arrow) portion in the diagram?

a. Genetic material such as DNA or RNA
b. Hydrolytic enzymes such as β-lactamases
c. Lipid A
d. LPS
e. Teichoic acid

**40.** A 55-year-old British teacher presents with weight-loss, weakness, muscle atrophy, and declining cognitive function. Her history reveals that her favorite meal is soup made with cow brain, which she has eaten almost every week since she was 10 years old. She is suspected to suffer from bovine spongiform encephalopathy. In comparing viruses with prions, which of the following statements is most likely true?

a. Both prions and viruses contain some form and quantity of nucleic acid, either DNA, RNA, or both
b. Both viruses and prions upon infection induce an antibody response in the host
c. Both viruses and prions upon infection induce an inflammatory response in the host
d. Conventional viruses are rapidly inactivated by ultraviolet light or heat, whereas prions are not
e. Both viral and prion proteins are encoded by viral genes

**41.** Over 200 isoniazid-resistant strains of *Mycobacterium tuberculosis* isolated from different patients in the northwestern region of Russia are screened by a PCR-restriction fragment length polymorphism assay. This analysis reveals a 93.6% prevalence of a specific G to C mutation in the *katG* in strains from patients with both newly and previously diagnosed cases of tuberculosis. Which of the following best describes the type of mutation that resulted in isoniazid resistance in these strains?

a. Inversion
b. Missense
c. Nonsense
d. Transition
e. Transversion

**42.** Posaconazole (SCH56592) is a potent, novel, broad-spectrum triazole in Phase III trials. Both *in vitro* and *in vivo* testing have demonstrated that posaconazole is more effective than fluconazole against *Candida* spp. and *Aspergillus* spp. Seven closely related isolates of *Candida albicans* exhibited progressive decreases in susceptibility to both posaconazole and itraconazole. Four of the isolates had amino acid changes, which were previously associated with azole resistance. Which of the following best describes the type of mutation that has resulted in decreased sensitivity to Posaconazole resistance in these strains?

a. Inversion
b. Missense
c. Nonsense
d. Transition
e. Transversion

**43.** A patient presents to the emergency room with vomiting, diarrhea, high fever, and delirium. Upon physical exam, you notice large, painful buboes, and disseminated intravascular coagulation. Laboratory diagnosis of aspirate taken from the bubo reveals a gram-negative rod with bipolar staining resembling a safety pin. Which of the following antibiotics is most appropiate as part of your immediate treatment?

a. Ceftazidine
b. Ceftriaxone
c. Penicillin
d. Streptomycin
e. Vancomycin

**44.** A 3-year-old girl who has missed several scheduled immunizations presents to the emergency room with a high fever. She is irritable and has a stiff neck. Fluid from a spinal tap reveals 20,000 white blood cells per milliliter with 85% polymorphonuclear cells. Which of the following is the preferred third-generation cephalosporin with good activity against organisms of childhood meningitis?

a. Ceftazidine
b. Ceftriaxone
c. Penicillin
d. Streptomycin
e. Vancomycin

**45.** A patient presents to the emergency room with a progressive fever, cough, and general malaise. History determines that he works with sheep on a farm and had just been involved in wool harvesting. Which of the following antibiotics is most appropiate as part of your immediate treatment?

a. Ceftazidine
b. Ceftriaxone
c. Penicillin
d. Streptomycin
e. Vancomycin

**46.** During the course of his hospital stay, a severely burned 60-year-old male develops a rapidly disseminating bacterial infection. Small gram-negative rods that are oxidase positive are cultured from green pus taken from the burn tissue. Which of the following third-generation cephalosporin will most likely have the best primary activity against this etiologic agent?

a. Ceftazidine
b. Ceftriaxone
c. Penicillin
d. Streptomycin
e. Vancomycin

**47.** Laboratory results of a clinical specimen from a patient with hospital-acquired pneumonia reveal the presence of *Staphylococcus aureus* with a methicillin-resistant plasmid. Which of the following drugs is the best immediate treatment?

a. Ceftazidine
b. Ceftriaxone
c. Penicillin
d. Streptomycin
e. Vancomycin

**48.** Antibiotics that inhibit dihydrofolic acid reductase in bacteria up to 50,000 times more than in mammalian cells is represented by which of the following agents?

a. Amdinocillin
b. Amphotericin
c. Chloramphenicol
d. Penicillin
e. Trimethoprim

**49.** An 18-year-old college freshman presents with fever of 103°F, headache, right flank pain, nausea and vomiting, and urinary frequency with hematuria and dysuria. Renal ultrasound demonstrates a right urinary stone with right hydronephrosis. Which of the following antibiotics binds to PBP-2 and is the most appropriate treatment option?

a. Amdinocillin
b. Amphotericin
c. Chloramphenicol
d. Penicillin
e. Trimethoprim

**50.** A 75-year-old African American male with neurogenic bladder presents to the emergency room with hypertension, fever up to 104.6°F, and nausea and vomiting. The urine from his foley catheter gives a positive culture for *Enterococcus faecalis*. Which of the following antibiotics inhibits the final peptide bond between d-alanine and glycine and is the most appropriate treatment for this patient?

a. Amdinocillin
b. Amphotericin
c. Chloramphenicol
d. Penicillin
e. Trimethoprim

**51.** A patient with leukemia has a chest CT finding that suggests aspergillosis. Which of the following antimicrobial binds sterols and alters membrane permeability, and would most likely be used in this patient's treatment?

a. Amdinocillin
b. Amphotericin
c. Chloramphenicol
d. Penicillin
e. Trimethoprim

**52.** A 10-week-old infant is diagnosed with meningitis. A lumbar puncture reveals numerous neutrophils and gram-positive rods. She is admitted to the hospital and is throught to be allergic to β-lactams. Which of the following antibiotics attaches to 50S ribosome, inhibits peptidyl transferase, and would most likely be used to treat this patient?

a. Amdinocillin
b. Amphotericin
c. Chloramphenicol
d. Penicillin
e. Trimethoprim

**Item 53–57**

An outbreak of diarrhea is thought to be related to a group of vendors who were selling hotdogs at a local carnival. Stool cultures are positive for *Salmonella* in almost all the patients. To determine the relatedness of the strains and determine the source of the infection, DNA is isolated from all the strains. The following diagram illustrates the amplification of a conserved region of the DNA by PCR. There are at least four points in the PCR process (A–D) that are critical to the reaction.

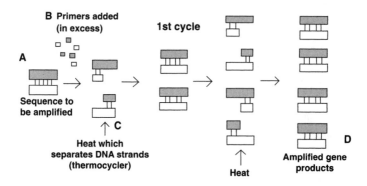

**53.** The Southern blot detection system for amplified PCR products fails to function. Which of the following would most likely be affected?

a. A
b. B
c. C
d. D

**54.** DNA does not hybridize with the primers. Which of the following would most likely be affected?

a. A
b. B
c. C
d. D

**55.** The laboratory observes a series of false-positive results. Which of the following processes is most likely faulty?

a. A
b. B
c. C
d. D

**56.** The DNA strands fail to reanneal. Which of the following processes is most likely faulty?

a. A
b. B
c. C
d. D

**57.** The laboratory observes a series of false-negative results. Which of the following processes is most likely faulty?

a. A
b. B
c. C
d. D

**58.** *Neiserria meningitidis*, group B, is identified as the cause of a local meningitis outbreak in a military training camp. This organism is characterized by which one of the following?

a. γ-Glutamyl polypeptide
b. Hyaluronic acid
c. Outer-membrane proteins
d. Repeating polysaccharide capsule of glucose and glucuronic acid
e. Sialic acid polymers

**59.** Group A streptococci (GAS) causes a wide range of infection presentations, ranging from skin lesions to toxic shock syndrome. GAS are characterized by which of the following?

a. γ-Glutamyl polypeptide
b. Hyaluronic acid
c. Outer-membrane proteins
d. Repeating polysaccharide capsule of glucose and glucuronic acid
e. Sialic acid polymers

**60.** Bacterial endotoxins may be inducers of inflammation by activating complement, resulting in hypotension. Bacterial LPS is characterized by which of the following?

a. Glycolipids (waxes)
b. Ketodeoxyoctulonate (KDO)
c. Phospholipid
d. Repeating polysaccharide capsule of glucose and glucuronic acid
e. Ribitol teichoic acid

**61.** Mycobacteria are stained by the acid-fast technique because their cell walls are characterized by which of the following?

a. Glycolipids (waxes)
b. KDO
c. Phospholipid
d. Repeating polysaccharide capsule of glucose and glucuronic acid
e. Ribitol teichoic acid

**62.** *Bacillus anthracis* is frequently described as a bioterrorism agent. Among its virulence factors can be found toxins (PA, EF, LF) as well as capsules which consist of which of the following materials?

a. Poly-D-glutamic acid
b. Hyaluronic acid
c. Outer-membrane proteins
d. Repeating polysaccharide capsule of glucose and glucuronic acid
e. Sialic acid polymers

**63.** *S. pneumoniae* cause significant morbidity and mortality due to capsular virulence factors. These capsules (55 antigenic types) are characterized by which of the following?

a.  γ-Glutamyl polypeptide
b.  Hyaluronic acid
c.  Outer-membrane proteins
d.  Repeating polysaccharide capsule of glucose and glucuronic acid
e.  Sialic acid polymers

# Physiology and Molecular Microbiology

## Answers

**1. The answer is d.** (*Levinson, pp 67–70. Ryan, pp 196–198.*) The structural integrity of the β-lactam ring in penicillins is essential for their antimicrobial activity. Many resistant strains of staphylococci produce an enzyme, penicillinase, that cleaves the β-lactam ring at the carbon-nitrogen bond. Other organisms, including certain coliform bacteria, produce an amidase enzyme that inactivates penicillin by disrupting the bond between the radical and nitrogen in the free amino group (1 in the diagram).

**2. The answer is e.** (*Ryan, pp 28–29.*) Almost no important nutrients enter the bacterial cell through simple diffusion, an exception being carbon dioxide and oxygen. Some diffusion, however, is facilitated by specific protein carriers. Most transport, except simple diffusion, is energy-dependent, particularly in gram-negative bacteria. Group translocation occurs in the absence of oxygen. For example, a simple carbohydrate such as glucose is phosphorylated enzymatically and is then transported into the cell.

**3. The answer is d.** (*Ryan, p 29.*) Siderophores such as aerobactin and enterobactin are chelators that trap iron $Fe^{3+}$. This Fe-chelator complex is actually transported inside the cell. Transferrin and lactoferrin are iron-binding proteins found in blood and milk. Ferric or iron oxide is rust, and LPS is a microbial cell-wall constituent.

**4. The answer is c.** (*Levinson, pp 6–7, 133–134. Ryan, p 19.*) The periplasm is the space between the outer membrane and the plasma membrane of bacteria. The periplasmic space in *E. coli* has been shown to contain a number of proteins, sugars, amino acids, and inorganic ions. Ethylenediaminetetraacetic acid (EDTA) is a chelating agent that disrupts the cell walls of gram-negative bacteria.

**5–6. The answers are 5-e, 6-d.** (*Levinson, pp 15–16, 100–102. Ryan, p 31.*) Oxygen, when it is metabolized, gives rise to hydrogen peroxide ($H_2O_2$)

and superoxide-anion ($O_2$). Both of these by products are extremely toxic to cells. Peroxide is produced by many bacteria, particularly facultative anaerobes that use flavoprotein intermediates. $H_2O_2$ is degraded by peroxidases, as illustrated in equation 2. Superoxide is detoxified by a critical enzyme known as *superoxide dismutase*. Such metabolism also results in $H_2O_2$ production (equation 1). *Peroxidase* and *catalase* are often used interchangeably to describe $H_2O_2$ reactions. However, in equation 2 when the $H_2A$ reactant is another $H_2O_2$ molecule, the enzyme is known as *catalase*. If $H_2A$ is another intermediate, then the enzyme is known as *peroxidase*.

**7. The answer is c.** (*Levinson, pp 100–102. Ryan, p 31.*) Superoxide dismutase is an enzyme found in both prokaryotic and eukaryotic cells that can survive in an environment of $O_2$. Lack of this enzyme, as well as peroxidase and catalase, ensures that a bacterium will not grow in the presence of $O_2$. Absence of these enzymes is not related to virulence, although ability to survive in an $O_2$-rich atmosphere may impart certain benefits to the proliferation of bacteria in the human host. Aminoglycosides and trimethoprim-sulfa drugs are never active against anaerobes.

**8–9.** The answers are 8-a, 9-d. (*Ryan, pp 251–255.*) Although traditional PCR had many advantages in speeding up the process of detecting the presence/absence of DNA/RNA in a sample, it had many limitations, with end-point detection being its largest problem. End-point detection involves the need for running agarose gel electrophoresis of the PCR product to visualize the presence/absence of DNA/RNA in a sample. This is time consuming, messy, and, overall, not ideal in the clinical setting. This led to the development of an enhanced modality known as *real-time PCR.*

With the advent of real-time PCR, many of the limitations of traditional PCR have been overcome. Real-time PCR allows for the detection of PCR amplification during the early phases of the PCR reaction and therefore avoids the need for gel electrophoresis, thus minimizing time to detection. The same stage cycling (denaturation, annealing, extension) used in traditional PCR is also utilized in the real-time PCR system. The difference, however, exists in the dependence of real-time PCR on a fluorescent reporter for the detection and quantitation of target DNA. This reporter signal increases in direct proportion to the amount of PCR product (amplicon) in a reaction. By recording the amount of fluorescence emission at each cycle, it is possible to monitor the PCR during the exponential phase where the first significant increase in the amount of PCR product correlates to the initial amount of target template. There are two general methods for the quantitative detection of the amplicon: (1) fluorescent probes (FAM, TAMRA, TET, ROX, and the like) or (2) DNA-binding agents (SYBR-green I, ethidium bromide, and the like).

SYBR-green is a dye that binds the minor groove of double-stranded DNA (dsDNA). When SYBR-green binds to dsDNA, the intensity of the fluorescent emissions increases. As more dsDNA amplicons are produced, the SYBR-green signal will increase, allowing for real-time analysis while the PCR is running.

Real-time PCR is a powerful improvement over the traditional PCR system and can be applied to such investigations as (1) viral quantitation, (2) quantitation of gene expression, (3) array verification, (4) drug therapy efficacy, (5) DNA damage measurement, (6) quality control and assay validation, (7) pathogen detection (rapid and accurate), and (8) genotyping. A real-time PCR, in addition to requiring the same ingredients as a regular PCR (i.e., specimen/template DNA, forward primer, reverse primer, polymerase [Taq], dNTPs, MgCl$_2$, hepes buffer, H$_2$O), also requires the presence of a fluorescent reporter such as SYBR-green I. The diagram represented in question 9 was obtained using a Smart Cycler II real-time PCR machine purchased from Cepheid. Sigmoidal-shaped curves indicate amplification in vitro and, hence, presence of *N. gonorrhoeae* and HSV-2 in the collected clinical sample. Horizontal lines represent no amplification and the absence of *T. pallidum*, *H. ducreyi*, and *C. trachomatis* in the obtained clinical sample. Real-time PCR is becoming increasingly important in the clinical setting for rapid and sensitive identification of pathogens from clinically obtained samples, and thus should be a familiar process to every health care professional.

**10. The answer is c.** (*Levinson, pp 33, 117–118. Ryan, p 22.*) Bacteria may shift rapidly between the fimbriated (fim +) and the nonfimbriated (fim −) states. Fimbriae function as adhesions to specific surfaces and, consequently, play a major role in pathogenesis. Lack of fimbriae prevents colonization of the mucosal surface by the bacterium.

**11. The answer is d.** (*Levinson, pp 135–137, 475s. Ryan, pp 353, 362–363.*) Region 1 (the Oantigenic side chain of LPS is responsible for the many serotypes of *Salmonella*. A mutant of *Salmonella* deficient in region 1 is not identified as a "newport," at least by virtue of its somatic antigen; biochemical identification of this mutant would be *S. enteritidis.* Loss of region 1 does not affect genus and species classification of *Salmonella.* Recently, however, it has been recommended that *Salmonella* be referred to by genus and serovar, that is, *Salmonella newport* or *Salmonella* serovar *newport.*

**12. The answer is c.** (*Levinson, pp 8, 67–70. Ryan, pp 36, 196.*) Transpeptidases or PBPs combine with penicillin to keep the final cross-linking step in the synthesis of peptidoglycan in the cell wall. All of the other choices are involved in polymerization processes. Examples of polymerization include the cell membrane (bactoprenol) and synthesis of DNA and RNA.

**13. The answer is b.** (*Levinson, pp 12–13. Ryan, pp 24–25.*) Dipicolinic acid, formed in the synthesis of diaminopimelate (DAP), is a prominent component of bacterial spores but is not found in vegetative cells or eukaryotic appendages or fimbrial structures. The calcium salt of dipicolinic acid apparently plays an important role in stabilizing spore proteins, but its mechanism of action is unknown. Dipicolinic acid synthetase is an enzyme unique to bacterial spores.

**14–16. The answers are 14-a, 15-b, 16-c.** (*Levinson, p 15. Ryan, pp 41–42.*) Bacterial growth curves are multiphasic. The lag phase is characterized by lack of growth but not necessarily metabolic activity. The bacteria are "adjusting" to their new environment. Depending on the bacteria, the temperature, nutrients, and pH, the microorganisms start dividing after a few hours and grow logarithmically for 12–18 hours. Toxins accumulate in the medium and nutrients become limiting. Oxygen and $CO_2$ are usually not limiting, as the gases freely diffuse into the growing culture. When death and growth of cells are equal, the stationary phase occurs. The death phase is characterized by a death rate that is more rapid than the growth rate. An antibiotic that inhibits protein synthesis would be optimally active in a rapidly dividing culture where proteins are being rapidly synthesized, that is, the logarithmic phase. Bacteria introduced into the human host may undergo similar phases of growth. However, other factors such as host defenses play a major role in limiting logarithmic growth, as does accumulation of toxic by-products as might occur in a closed-space infection such as an abscess.

**17. The answer is c.** (*Levinson, pp 75–76. Ryan, pp 215–216.*) Ideally, antibiotics should attack a microbial structure or function not found in human cells. Except for mitomycin, all the antibiotics listed in the question interfere with cell-wall synthesis in bacteria. Mitomycin inhibits DNA synthesis in both mammalian and microbial systems; viral DNA synthesis, however, is relatively resistant to mitomycin.

**18–19. The answers are 18-b, 19-d.** (Levinson, pp 7–8. Ryan, pp 16, 232–233.) First described in 1884 by a Danish physician, Hans Christian Gram, the Gram stain has proved to be one of the most useful diagnostic laboratory procedures in microbiology and medicine. The Gram stain procedure is characterized by the following steps: (1) *fixation* of the bacteria to the slide, (2) crystal violet (acridine dye) treatment, (3) iodine treatment, (4) *decolorization* using alcohol/acetone wash, and (4) *counterstaining* using safranin. Gram-positive bacteria have thick outer walls with no lipids, whereas gram-negative bacteria have a thin wall and an outer membrane. The difference between gram-positive and gram-negative organisms is in the cell-wall permeability to these complexes on treatment with mixtures of acetone and alcohol solvents. Thus, gram-positive bacteria retain purple iodine-dye complexes, whereas gram-negative bacteria do not retain these complexes when decolorized using an alcohol/acetone wash. If the iodine treatment step is omitted during the Gram stain process, the purple iodine-dye complexes will not form. The crystal violet will wash away during the alcohol/acetone decolorization washing step and all cells will appear *red.* Gram staining of pus or fluids along with clinical findings can guide the management of an infection before culture results are available in the clinical setting.

**20. The answer is e.** (Levinson, p 6. Ryan, pp 19, 21.) A porin is a protein trimer with each subunit containing a pore with a diameter of 1 nm. Porins function in outer-membrane (OM) permeability. While porins are known to permit the transfer of small molecules across the OM, specific porins may also influence the diffusion of layer molecules. Also, porins can regulate the passage of many antimicrobial drugs such as ampicillin. Depending on charge, porins may also repel certain molecules, such as bile salts found in the intestinal environment.

**21. The answer is d.** (Levinson, pp 24, 170–172. Ryan, pp 434–437.) The serologic diagnosis of Lyme disease is fraught with difficulty. Enzyme immunoassay (EIA) may be insensitive in the early stages of disease and may lack specificity in advanced stages. Western blot analysis of the antibody is the confirmatory test for Lyme disease, but it, too, is not 100% sensitive and specific. The Western blot test detects antibodies to proteins and glycoproteins of *Borrelia burgdorferi*. Not all of these proteins are specific for the organism. For example, antibodies to Gp66 may reflect a cross-reaction, as many gram-negative bacteria have similar glycoproteins. For this reason, a Western blot showing only antibodies to Gp66 is thought to be a nonspecific immune response.

**22. The answer is b.** (*Ryan, pp 251–253.*) DNA polymerase isolated from the hot springs thermophilic bacterium named *T. aquaticus* is essential for the PCR process because of its stability at high temperatures (95°C). While the *E. coli* enzyme can be used, the enzyme itself becomes denatured, fewer cycles are possible, and nonspecific reactions occur because of hybridization of primers to nontarget DNA. The use of Taq polymerase allows DNA copying at 72°C rather than 37°C, which further reduces nonspecific hybridization.

**23–25. The answers are 23-b, 24-d, 25-e.** (*Ryan, pp 251–255.*) The PCR has revolutionized the detection of infectious microorganisms, particularly those that are difficult to grow. During their normal practice, physicians will usually not be required to design a PCR test, but they should know some of the design elements of PCR so that they might better understand the results from these widely used tests.

One of the major problems of PCR in the past was contamination from extraneous nucleic acid. There are several ways to prevent contamination and the resulting falsely positive results. They include the use of separate laboratories, hoods, gloves, and surface disinfectants. The most effective method, however, is the use of internal sterilizing agents such as uracil N-glycosyls (UNG). These agents cross-link extraneous DNA so that the product cannot be amplified. Primers can now be purchased from a catalog and their sequence obtained online. Primers are easily synthesized, must be complementary to sequences on the bacterial chromosome, and when coupled to such sequences must promote replication. The specificity of PCR is a function of choosing a primer pair that is unique to the organism that you wish to detect. The PCR process is best explained by the "needle in the haystack" analogy. One needle in a haystack is difficult to find. However, if one needle becomes a million needles, then detection is easy. The same is true for nucleic acids. The amplicons (amplified nucleic acids) can be detected by a number of methods because they are so plentiful. These methods include specific staining with ethidium bromide of a gel containing these amplicons, and Southern blotting of the amplicons "tags" them so that they can be seen on photographic film. Amplicons are also bound to solid phases and detected with labeled enzymes or an instrument that reads a fluorescent tag. Microscopy is not used.

**26. The answer is c.** (*Levinson, p 8–9. Ryan, p 19.*) The organisms illustrated in the question are spheroplasts of *E. coli*. Lysozyme clears the β-1-4-glycosidic bond between N-acetylmuramic acid and N-acetylglucosamine. Spheroplasts are bacteria with cell walls that have been partially removed by the action of lysozyme or penicillin. Ordinarily, with disintegration of the walls, the cells undergo lysis; however, in a hypertonic medium, the cells persist and assume a spherical configuration. Endospores are formed by gram-positive bacteria in the genera *Bacillus* and *Clostridium*. It has also been shown that for *E. coli* and other gram-negative rods, exposure to minimal concentrations of antibiotics does not rupture the cell wall but promotes elongation of the cell by inhibiting the division cycle.

**27. The answer is d.** (*Ryan, pp 252–253.*) Gene cloning is a basic step in virtually every genetic engineering process. First, the source DNA is isolated and cut into small pieces and then attached to a cloning vector with DNA ligase. The cloning vectors are inserted into the host organism (usually a bacterium), and then the cloned DNA is isolated, identified, and purified. Amplification of source DNA is not a necessary step.

**28. The answer is d.** (*Ryan, pp 251–255.*) Nucleic acid probes, either DNA or RNA, are commonly used in clinical and research microbiology laboratories. These complementary pieces of nucleic acid bind to genes or gene parts of interest and are detected by their label, which may be either radioactive or nonradioactive. Probes, in general, are more sensitive than traditional growth-dependent methods, particularly for those microorganisms that either cannot be cultured or grow very slowly.

**29. The answer is e.** (*Ryan, pp 251–255.*) PCR is a widely used tool for amplification of small pieces of nucleic acid present in minute quantities.

Once the sequence to be amplified is known, a specific forward and reverse primer is added. The temperature is alternately raised and lowered up to 45–50 times in the presence of a heat-resistant DNA polymerase from *T. aquaticus.* The amplified gene product is then detected by one of a number of techniques such as cloning, direct hybridization, agarose gel electrophoresis, and southern hybridization.

**30–33. The answers are 30-d, 31-e, 32-c, 33-b.** *(Levinson, pp 67–77. Ryan, pp 35, 41–42, 194–199, 201–202, 204.)* Penicillin causes lysis of growing bacterial cells. Its antimicrobial effect stems from impairment of cell-wall synthesis. Because penicillin is bactericidal, the number of viable cells should fall immediately after introduction of the drug into the medium.

Both chloramphenicol and sulfonamides are bacteriostatic—that is, they retard cell growth without causing cell death. Chloramphenicol causes an immediate, reversible, bacteriostatic inhibition of protein synthesis. Sulfonamides, on the other hand, compete with para-aminobenzoic acid in the synthesis of folate; intracellular stores of folate are depleted gradually as the cells continue to grow.

The number of viable cells in a culture eventually will level off, even if no antibiotic is added to the environment. A key factor in this phenomenon is the limited availability of substrate.

**34–36. The answers are 34-e, 35-d, 36-b.** *(Levinson, pp 17–22. Ryan, pp 57–64.)* Transformation, transduction, and conjugation are critical processes in which DNA is transferred from one bacterium to another. Transformation, the passage of high-molecular-weight DNA from one bacterium to another, was first observed in pneumococci. Later studies have shown that, at least in *S. pneumoniae,* double-stranded DNA is "nicked" by a membrane-bound endonuclease, initiating DNA entry into the host cell. One of the nicked DNA strands is digested, and the other is integrated into the host genome. Transduction, which can affect many bacteria, is a process in which a fragment of donor chromosome is carried to a recipient cell by a temperate virus (bacteriophage). In generalized transduction, the phage virus can carry any segment of the donor chromosome; in restricted transduction, the phage carries only those chromosomal segments immediately adjacent to the site of prophage attachment. In conjugation, too, DNA is passed from one bacterium to another. However, instead of the transfer of soluble DNA, a small loop of DNA, called a *plasmid,* is passed between cells. Examples of plasmids are the sex factors and the resistance (R) factors.

**37. The answer is d.** (*Levinson, pp 15–16.*) Bacteria reproduce by binary fission and thus undergo exponential (logarithmic) growth. In this question, the chart indicates a doubling time for *E. coli* as 20 minutes. Therefore, after 2 hours there will be six doubling times. Using the equation $2^n$, where $n$ equals the number of generations, and remembering that we started with five *E. coli* cells in the start culture, we rewrite this equation after 2 hours as $5 \times 2^n$; thus, the number of *E. coli* cells in the culture after 2 hours is $5 \times 2^6 = 320$.

**38. The answer is a.** (*Levinson, p 48. Ryan, pp 305–306.*) Koch's postulates, formulated by Robert Koch in 1877, were an attempt to determine the cause of infectious disease. Simply stated, they consist of four statements: (1) A specific organism must be isolated from every diseased patient; (2) the organism must be isolated in vitro in pure culture; (3) when inoculated, the pure organism must cause the disease in a healthy, susceptible animal; and (4) the organism must be reisolated from the infected animal.

**39. The answer is b.** (*Levinson, pp 6–7. Ryan, pp 14–15, 18–21.*) The area indicated by the arrow in the diagram is known as the *periplasmic space,* which is the space between the plasma membrane and the outer membrane. This space contains many hydrolytic enzymes such as alkaline phosphatase, antibiotic-inactivating enzymes such as β-lactamases, and various binding proteins involved in chemotaxis and the active transport of solutes into the cell.

**40. The answer is d.** (*Levinson, pp 189–190, 308–312. Ryan, pp 80, 624–628.*) Prions are infectious particles that are composed solely of protein (i.e., they contain no detectable nucleic acid). On the other hand, viruses contain both protein and nucleic acid. Prions give rise to a number of "slow" diseases known as transmissible spongiform encepalopathies such as Creutzfeldt-Jakob disease in humans, bovine spongiform encephalopathy (BSE) in cows, and scrapie in sheep. Prions are unusually resistant to ultraviolet irradiation, alcohol, formalin, boiling, proteases, and nucleases. They can be inactivated by prolonged exposure to steam autoclaving or 1N or 2N NaOH. This has strong implications in the sterilization procedure used for certain medical instruments. The following table is an excellent comparison between conventional viruses and prions.

| COMPARISON OF PRIONS AND CONVENTIONAL VIRUSES | | |
|---|---|---|
| Feature | Prions | Conventional Viruses |
| Particle contains nucleic acid | No | Yes |
| Particle contains protein | Yes, encoded by cellular genes | Yes, encoded by viral genes |
| Inactivated rapidly by UV light or heat | No | Yes |
| Appearance in electron microscope | Filamentous rods (amyloid-like) | Icosahedral or helical symmetry |
| Infection induces antibody | No | Yes |
| Infection induces inflammation | No | Yes |

Reprinted, with permission, from Levinson W, Jawetz E. Medical Microbiology and Immunology, 7e. New York: McGraw-Hill, 2002.

**41–42. The answers are 41-e, 42-b.** *(Levinson, pp 17–22. Ryan, pp 54–57, Mokrousov et al. Antimicrob Agents Chemother. 2002 May; 46(5): 1417–1424, Li et al. Journal of Antimicrobial Chemotherapy (2004) 53, 74–80.)* Mutations result from three types of molecular changes, namely, base substitution mutation, frame shift mutation, and transposon or insertion sequences causing mutations. Inversion mutations are caused by insertion sequences (ISs) or IS-like elements. Missense mutation refers to base substitution resulting in a codon that causes a different amino acid to be inserted. Nonsense mutation refers to base substitution generating a termination codon that prematurely stops protein synthesis. Transition mutations are the replacement of a pyrimidine (C, T) by a pyrimidine or a purine (A, G) by a purine. Transversion mutations are the replacement of a purine by a pyrimidine or pyrimidine by a purine.

**43–47. The answers are 43-d, 44-b, 45-c, 46-a, 47-e.** *(Levinson, pp 154–155, 80, 119–121, 144, 70, 103–106. Ryan, pp 198, 220–221, 269–270, 305–307, 484–488.)* The patient in question 43 is infected with *Yersinia pestis* and has bubonic plague. Ceftriaxone or cefotaxime are preferred in the treatment of childhood meningitis because they have the highest activity against the three major causes, namely, *Haemophilus influenzae, N. meningitidis,* and *S. pneumoniae.* The patient in question 45 has woolsorter's disease (inhalation anthrax) from contaminated wool on the farm where he works. Of the third-generation cephalosporins, only ceftazidine is consistently active against *P. aeroginosa.* Finally, the patient in question 47 has acquired a methicillin-resistant *S. aureus* (MRSA) infection, against which vancomycin may be effective. However, *S. aureus* strains are emerging with decreased susceptibility to vancomycin.

**48–52.  The answers are 48-e, 49-a, 50-d, 51-b, 52-c.** *(Levinson, pp 67–81. Ryan, pp 195–198, 201–202, 204, 643–644.)* The antibiotics in these questions have significantly different modes of action. Recent evidence suggests that while penicillin inhibits the final cross-linking of the cell wall, it also binds to penicillin-binding proteins and inhibits certain key enzymes involved in cell-wall synthesis. The mechanism is complex. Amdinocillin, although classified as a penicillin, selectively binds to PBP-2. Binding to PBP-2 results in aberrant cell-wall elongation and spherical forms, seen when *E. coli,* for example, is exposed to mecillinam.

Because amphotericin binds to sterols (such as ergosterol, a compound of fungal membrane) in the cell membrane, its range of activity is predictable; that is, it is effective against microorganisms that contain sterol in the cell membrane (such as molds, yeasts, and certain amebas). These polyene antibiotics cause reorientation of sterols in the membrane, and membrane structure is altered to the extent that permeability is affected. If sterol synthesis is blocked in fungi, then amphotericin is not effective. This occurs when fungi are exposed to miconazole, another antifungal antibiotic.

Chloramphenicol can be either bacteriocidal or bacteriostatic, depending on the organism. It is bacteriostatic against organisms such as *S. typhi,* but is bacteriocidal against encapsulated organisms that cause meningitis such as *H. influenzae, S. pneumoniae,* and *N. meningitidis.* Bacterial ribosomes are spherical particles. Protein synthesis takes place on the ribosome by a complex process involving various ribosomal subunits, tRNA, and mRNA. Chloramphenicol, in contrast to the aminoglycosides and tetracycline, attaches to the 50S ribosome subunit. The enzyme peptidyl transferase, found in the 50S subunit, is inhibited. Removal of the inhibition—in this case, chloramphenicol—results in full activity of the enzyme.

Trimethoprim (TMP), a diaminopyrimidine, is a folic acid antagonist. Although TMP is commonly used in combination with sulfa drugs, its mode of action is distinct. TMP is structurally similar to the pteridine portion of dihydrofolate and prevents the conversion of folic acid to tetrahydrofolic acid by inhibition of dihydrofolate reductase. Fortunately, this enzyme in humans is relatively insensitive to TMP.

**53–57.** The answers are 53-d, 54-c, 55-a, 56-c, 57-b. (*Ryan, pp 251–255.*) The process of PCR is complicated, and its steps are interrelated. A number of steps in the process can markedly affect the results of clinical testing. For example, the detection of amplified products is essential in order to determine whether target nucleic acid was present in the specimen. Product can be detected by staining of the gel that separates the products, Southern blot (a radioactive procedure), or an ELISA-like capture method. A failure of this production step prevents detection of product.

One of the essential parts of the PCR process is the thermal cycling of the reaction. If the reaction is not heated, primer DNA will not hybridize with the target sequences. Nor will the strands reanneal if the mixture is not cooled. Failure of the thermocycler could cause such a problem.

False-positive results are usually due to contamination of the reaction by foreign DNA. In such a case, the foreign DNA sequences are amplified even if the target sequences are not present.

There are a number of reasons why PCR would be falsely negative, but a prime reason is failure to choose the right primer sets. Suboptimum detection of amplified products is another. Ethidium bromide staining of the PCR gel is less sensitive than detection of the products by Southern blot.

**58–63. The answers are 58-e, 59-b, 60-b, 61-a, 62-a, 63-d.** (*Levinson, pp 6–7, 107–111, 45–48, 7–8, 119–121, 11. Ryan, pp 19–20, 164, 276, 288–293, 305–307, 329–333, 439–442.*) Bacteria have a variety of components; some are unique to certain genera and species, others are characteristic of all bacteria. All bacteria have peptidoglycan in their cell walls, although the peptidoglycan layer is much thinner in gram-negative than in gram-positive bacteria. In gram-positive bacteria, teichoic acids, polysaccharides, and peptidoglycolipids are covalently attached to the peptidoglycans. While *Mycobacterium* also has peptidoglycan, up to 40% of the cell wall may be a waxy glycolipid that is responsible for the "acid fastness" of *Mycobacterium* and *Nocardia,* an aerobic actinomycete. Bacterial LPS, also known as *endotoxin,* is found only in gram-negative bacteria. Not only is it a toxic macromolecule, but it also imparts serologic specificity to some gram-negative bacteria such as *Salmonella* and *E. coli*. A core polysaccharide of several sugars is linked to Lipid A by KDO.

Capsules are found in both gram-positive and gram-negative bacteria. With the exception of those found in *Bacteroides fragilis*, capsules are not in and of themselves toxic but rather are antiphagocytic and are immunologic (or serologic) determinants. Some examples of capsular components are the following:

1. Sialic acid polymers are found in group B *N. meningitidis*. This identical polymer is also found in *E. coli* K1.
2. Group A streptococci in the early stages of growth have hyaluronic acid capsules. The capsule, however, is rapidly destroyed by the organism's own hyaluronidase.
3. *B. anthracis*, the causative agent of anthrax, is the only bacterium to possess a polypeptide capsule that is a polymer of glutamic acid.
4. *S. pneumoniae* type 3 has a repeating polysaccharide capsule of glucose and glucuronic acid.

# Virology

## Questions

**DIRECTIONS:** Each question below contains four or more suggested responses. Select the **one best** response to each question.

**64.** An HIV-positive patient has progressed from fatigue, rash, nausea, and night sweats symptoms to occasional but defined opportunistic infections. He inquires as to what can be done to predict his chances of developing symptomatic AIDS. Which of the following tests would be most useful?

a. CD4 lymphocyte count
b. HIV antibody test
c. HIV p24 antigen
d. HIV RT PCR
e. Neopterin

**65.** A 9-year-old male presents with fever and nonspecific symptoms followed by a distinctive rash on the cheeks (slapped cheek). Which of the following viruses is the most likely cause of this disease and has been associated with transient aplastic crises in persons with sickle cell disease?

a. *Herpes simplex*
b. Parvovirus B19
c. Rubella
d. Rubeola
e. Varicella-zoster

**66.** A 20-year-old female presents to her physician with a low-grade fever, headache, and painful genital lesions. Culture detects herpes simplex virus (HSV). Which of the following statements best describes infection with this common human pathogen?

a. Infection with type 1 virus is most common
b. Initial infection usually occurs by intestinal absorption of the virus
c. It can be reactivated by emotional disturbances or prolonged exposure to sunlight
d. It rarely recurs in a host who has a high antibody titer
e. The central nervous system (CNS) and visceral organs are usually involved

**67.** Highly active antiretroviral therapy (HAART) became available in 1996, utilizing azidothymidine (AZT), dideoxyinosine (DDI), and saquinavir or similar agents. Use of these three drugs inhibits which of the following viral processes?

a.   All membrane synthesis
b.   gp120 formation
c.   p24 antibody expression
d.   Reverse transcriptase, protease
e.   RNase, DNase

**68.** An HIV-positive patient, prior to being treated with AZT, DDI, and saquinavir, has a CD4 lymphocyte count and an HIV RNA viral load test done. Results are as follows:

CD4: 50 CD4 lymphocytes per $\mu$L
HIV RNA: 100,000 copies per mL

Which of the following statements best describes this patient?

a.   This patient is no longer in danger of opportunistic infection
b.   The 5-year prognosis is excellent
c.   The patient's HIV screening test is most likely negative
d.   The patient is not infectious
e.   The viral load of 100,000 copies per milliliter suggests that the patient will respond to triple therapy

**69.** An HIV-positive patient with a viral load of 100,000 copies of HIV RNA/milliliter and a total CD4 count of 50 is at increased risk for a number of infectious diseases. For which of the following diseases is the patient at no more added risk than an immunocompetent host?

a.   Herpes simplex virus
b.   Kaposi sarcoma
c.   Mycobacterial disease
d.   Pneumococcal pneumonia
e.   Pneumocystic pneumonia

**70.** A 19-year-old college student presents to the student health clinic complaining of sore throat, fever, swollen neck lymph nodes, and malaise of several days. Viral capsid antibody (IgM) tests positive, indicating infectious mononucleosis. This potentially debilitating viral disorder is characterized by which of the following statements?

a. Affected persons respond to treatment with the production of heterophil antibodies
b. It is caused by a rhabdovirus
c. It is most prevalent in children less than 14 years old
d. Ribavirin is the treatment of choice
e. The causative pathogen is an Epstein-Barr virus (EBV)

**71.** During a medical checkup for a new insurance policy, a 60-year-old grandmother is found to be positive in the enzyme-linked immunosorbent assay (ELISA) screening test for antibodies against HIV-1. She has no known risk factors for exposure to the virus. Which of the following is the most appropriate next step?

a. Immediately begin therapy with azidothymidine
b. Perform the screening test a second time
c. Request that a blood culture be done by the lab
d. Tell the patient that she is likely to develop AIDS
e. Test the patient for *Pneumocystis carinii* infection

**72.** Patients in an outbreak of arbovirus disease on a Caribbean island present with a variety of symptoms, including encephalitis, hemorrhagic fever, or fever with myalgia. Which of the following is a characteristic of arboviruses?

a. Are closely related to Parvoviruses
b. Are transmitted by insect vectors
c. Are treatable with antiviral chemotherapy
d. Are usually resistant to ether
e. Usually cause symptomatic infection in humans

**73.** Recombinant interferon-α (IFN-α) is the currently approved therapy for patients who are chronically infected with hepatitis B virus (HBV) or hepatitis C virus (HCV). IFN was originally described in chicken embryo cells infected with influenza viruses. Which of the following statements best describes IFN's suspected mode of action as an antiviral reagent?

a. It stimulates a cell-mediated immunity
b. It stimulates humoral immunity
c. Its direct antiviral action is related to the suppression of messenger RNA formation
d. Its action is related to the synthesis of a protein that inhibits translation or transcription
e. It alters the permeability of the cell membrane so that viruses cannot enter the cell

**74.** Coronaviruses are recognized by club-shaped surface glycoproteins that are 20 nm long and resemble solar coronas. A SARS outbreak in 2003 was characterized by serious respiratory illness and progressive respiratory failure. Which of the following is a characteristic ability of non–SARS coronaviruses?

a. Agglutinate human red blood cells
b. Cause common cold
c. Grow profusely at 50°C
d. Grow well in the usual cultured cell lines
e. Infect infants more frequently than adults

**75.** An elderly male patient with known chronic HBV status suddenly presents with acute hepatitis episodes. Serology confirms hepatitis D virus (HDV) coinfection. Which one of the following best describes the delta agent?

a. A hepatitis B mutant
b. A defective RNA virus
c. An incomplete hepatitis B virus
d. Hepatitis C
e. Related to hepatitis A virus

**76.** Which of the following antiviral agents is a purine nucleoside analogue that has shown promise with Lassa fever, influenza A and B, and respiratory syncytial virus (RSV)?

a. Amantadine
b. Acyclovir
c. Ribavirin
d. Rimantadine
e. Vidarabine

**77.** Enteric cytopathogenic human orphan viruses (echoviruses) appear worldwide and are more apt to be found in young patients. Family studies demonstrated the ease and high frequency of transmission. Which of the following body systems is the main target of echoviruses?

a. Bladder and urinary tract
b. Blood and lymphatic systems
c. Central nervous system
d. Intestinal tract
e. Respiratory system

**78.** A newborn infant presents with disseminated vesicular lesions and failure to thrive. Herpes simplex virus (HSV) is suspected, and laboratory confirmation is desired to justify antiviral chemotherapy. Which of the following is the most sensitive test for the diagnosis of HSV meningitis in a newborn infant?

a. Cerebrospinal fluid (CSF) protein analysis
b. HSV culture
c. HSV IgG antibody
d. HSV polymerase chain reaction
e. Tzanck smear

**79.** Acute hemorrhagic conjunctivitis (AHC) is a contagious ocular infection characterized by pain, swelling of the eyelids, and subconjunctival hemorrhages. AHC has been reported to be caused by which of the following viruses?

a. Coronavirus
b. Enterovirus
c. Reovirus
d. Respiratory synctial virus
e. Rhinovirus

**80.** A 10-year-old boy is taken to his pediatrician after experiencing fever, malaise, and anorexia followed by tender swelling of his parotid glands. Which of the following characterizes infection by this etiologic agent?

a. Is apt to recur periodically in many affected persons
b. Is maintained in a large canine reservoir
c. Is preventable by immunization
d. Usually produces severe systemic manifestations
e. Will usually cause mumps orchitis in postpubertal males

**81.** An otherwise healthy 65-year-old male was in a car accident and broke several ribs on the left side. Approximately 12 days later he developed a painful, well-circumscribed vesicular rash over the left rib cage that persisted for several weeks. The rash is most likely due to which of the following?

a. Primary infection with herpes B virus
b. Primary infection with herpes simplex virus type 1
c. Primary infection with herpes simplex virus type 2
d. Reactivation of latent Epstein-Barr virus
e. Reactivation of latent varicella-zoster virus

**82.** A 3-year-old child presents at the physician's office with symptoms of coryza, conjunctivitis, low-grade fever, and small, bluish-white ulcerations on the buccal mucosa opposite the lower molars. The causative agent of this disease belongs to which one of the following groups of viruses?

a. Adenovirus
b. Herpesvirus
c. Paramyxovirus
d. Picornavirus
e. Orthomyxovirus

**83.** One of the most common sexually transmitted diseases that may lead to cervical carcinoma has recently had a vaccine developed and approved for use, and should be given before sexual activity occurs. Which one of the following viruses is the basis for this vaccine?

a. Adenovirus
b. Cytomegalovirus
c. Epstein-Barr virus
d. Herpes simplex virus
e. Papillomavirus

**84.** Two siblings, ages 2 and 4, experienced fever, rhinitis, and pharyngitis that resulted in laryngotracheo bronchitis. Both had a harsh cough and hoarseness. Which of the following viruses is the leading cause of their syndrome?

a. Adenovirus
b. Group B coxsackievirus
c. Parainfluenza virus
d. Rhinovirus
e. Rotavirus

**85.** Which of the following statements is true regarding hepatitis E virus (HEV), a recently characterized but unclassified virus?

a. It is not a threat to the blood supply
b. It is a major cause of bloodborne hepatitis
c. It is prevalent in North America
d. It is a single-stranded DNA virus
e. The disease resembles hepatitis C

**86.** Meningitis is characterized by the acute onset of fever and stiff neck. Aseptic meningitis may be caused by a variety of microbial agents. During the initial 24 hours of the course of aseptic meningitis, an affected person's CSF is characterized by which of the following laboratory findings?

a. Decreased protein content
b. Elevated glucose concentration
c. Eosinophilia
d. Lymphocytosis
e. Polymorphonuclear leukocytosis

**87.** Infection with HDV (delta agent) can occur simultaneously with infection with HBV or in a carrier of HBV, because HDV is a defective virus that requires HBV for its replicative function. Which of the following serologic tests can be used to determine whether a patient with HDV is an HBV carrier?

a. HBsAg
b. HBc IgM
c. HBeAg
d. HBs IgM
e. HBs IgG

**88.** A nurse develops clinical symptoms consistent with hepatitis. She recalls sticking herself with a needle approximately 4 months before, after drawing blood from a patient. Serologic tests for HBsAg, antibodies to HBsAg, and hepatitis A virus (HAV) are all negative; however, she is positive for IgM core antibody. Which of the following characterizes the current health state of the nurse?

a. Does not have hepatitis B
b. Has hepatitis A
c. Has hepatitis C
d. Is in the late stages of hepatitis B infection
e. Is in the "window" (after the disappearance of HBsAg and before the appearance of anti–HBsAg)

**89.** A 62-year-old Florida fisherman forgot his insect repellent on a recent sporting trip. A week later, he presented to his physician with fever, chills, headache, and flu-like symptoms that progressed to possible CNS involvement. Control of the etiologic agent, associated with a high (50–70%) fatality rate, could be possible by eradication of which of the following?

a. Birds
b. Fleas
c. Horses
d. Mosquitoes
e. Ticks

**90.** Rhinoviruses are the most commonly recovered agents from people with mild upper respiratory illlnesses and have very brief incubation periods. These agents are primarily transmitted by which one of the following mechanisms?

a. Droplet aerosolization
b. Fecal-oral route
c. Fomites
d. Sexual activity
e. Vertical transmission (mother to child)

**91.** A 9-year-old schoolchild developed malaise, a low-grade fever, and a morbilliform rash that appeared on the same day. The rash started on the face and spread to the extremities. Which of the following statements best describes the etiologic agent causing this disease?

a. Incubation time is approximately 3–4 weeks
b. Measles (rubeola) and German measles (rubella) are caused by the same virus
c. Onset is abrupt, with cough, coryza, and fever lasts 3 days
d. Specific antibody in the serum does not prevent disease
e. Vesicular rashes are characteristic

**92.** A biopsy specimen is collected from the skin of the neck at the hairline of a patient and is stained with immunofluorescent reagents. Results demonstrate host intranuclear inclusions which are sharply demarkated, spherical, and less than 10 μm in diameter. Which of the following is the most likely diagnosis?

a. Aseptic meningitis
b. Congenital rubella
c. Infectious mononucleosis
d. Mumps
e. Rabies

**93.** Kuru is a fatal disease of certain New Guinea natives and is characterized by tremors and ataxia; Creutzfeldt-Jakob disease (CJD) is characterized by both ataxia and dementia. These diseases are thought to be caused by which of the following?

a. Cell wall—deficient bacteria
b. Environmental toxins
c. Flagellates
d. Prions
e. Slow viruses

**94.** Vaccinia virus vaccine was used to eliminate variola from the world population. Recent concerns about possible terrorist use of variola have resulted in new recommendations for use of the vaccine. According to recommendations issued by the U.S. Public Health Service, which of the following statements regarding vaccination against smallpox is true?

a. Children should be vaccinated before they begin school
b. Persons traveling abroad need not be vaccinated
c. Persons who have eczema should be vaccinated soon after diagnosis
d. Persons who have immune deficiencies should be vaccinated every 5 years
e. Pregnant women should be vaccinated in the first trimester

**95.** A 35-year-old man developed headache, nausea, vomiting, and sore throat 8 weeks after returning from a trip abroad. He eventually refused to drink water and had episodes of profuse salivation, difficulty in breathing, and hallucinations. Two days after the patient died of cardiac arrest, it was learned that he had been bitten by a dog while on his trip. Which of the following treatments, if given immediately after the dog bite, could have helped prevent this disease?

a. Bed rest
b. Interleukin 2
c. High-dose acyclovir
d. Broad-spectrum antibiotics
e. Vaccine specific for the etiologic agent

**96.** A patient who works in an industrial setting presents to his ophthalmologist with acute conjunctivitis, enlarged and tender preauricular nodes, and early stages of keratitis. The differential diagnosis should include infection with which of the following viruses?

a. Adenovirus
b. Epstein-Barr virus
c. Parvovirus
d. Respiratory syncytial virus
e. Varicella-zoster virus

**97.** A hospital worker is found to have hepatitis B surface antigen. Subsequent tests reveal the presence of e antigen as well. Which of the following best describes the worker?

a. Is infective and has active hepatitis
b. Is infective but does not have active hepatitis
c. Is not infective
d. Is evincing a biologic false-positive test for hepatitis
e. Has both hepatitis B and hepatitis C

**98.** Alphaviruses grow initially in capillary cells and macrophages, producing a viremia and causing fever, headaches, backaches, and flu-like symptoms. A secondary viremia may lead to brain, liver, skin, and vasculature infections. Which of the following diseases is caused by an alphavirus?

a. Dengue
b. Marburg virus disease
c. Saint Louis encephalitis
d. Western equine encephalitis
e. Yellow fever

**99.** Several antiviral compounds have been developed during the last decade. One such compound is ribavirin, a synthetic nucleoside structurally related to guanosine. Ribavirin therapy is FDA-approved for use against which of the following?

a. Group A coxsackievirus
b. Hepatitis B
c. Herpes simplex virus
d. Parvovirus
e. Respiratory syncytial virus

**100.** An immunocompromised person with a history of seizures has an MRI that reveals a temporal lobe lesion. Brain biopsy results show multinucleated giant cells with intranuclear inclusions. Which of the following is the most probable cause of the lesion?

a. Coxsackievirus
b. Hepatitis C virus
c. Herpes simplex virus
d. *Listeria monocytogenes*
e. Parvovirus

**101.** A 19-year-old college freshwoman seeks medical help for symptoms of headache, malaise, fatigue, and sore throat. She admits to attending multiple parties in the dorm. Her physician notes her enlarged lymph nodes and spleen. Which of the following procedures or clinical signs is most specific for the diagnosis of infectious mononucleosis caused by the Epstein-Barr virus (EBV)?

a. B-cell lymphocyte proliferation
b. Growth in tissue culture cells
c. Heterophile antibodies in serum
d. Laboratory diagnosis based on the presence of "atypical lymphocytes" and EBV-specific antibody
e. Lymphadenopathy and splenomegaly on physical examination

**102.** A 5-month-old infant, seen in the ER, presents with a fever and persistent cough with wheezing. Physical examination and a chest x-ray suggest pneumonia. Which of the following is most likely the cause of this infection?

a. Adenovirus
b. Coxsackievirus
c. Respiratory syncytial virus
d. Rhinovirus
e. Rotavirus

**103.** Which one of the following groups of people may be at increased risk for HIV infection?

a. Factory workers whose coworkers are HIV-positive
b. Foreign service employees who are hospitalized in Zaire for bleeding ulcers
c. Homosexual females
d. Members of a household in which there is a person who is HIV-positive
e. Receptionists at a hospital

**104.** An obstetrician sees a pregnant patient who was exposed to rubella virus in the 18th week of pregnancy. She does not remember getting a rubella vaccination. Which of the following is the best immediate course of action?

a.  Administer rubella immune globulin
b.  Administer rubella vaccine
c.  Order a rubella antibody titer to determine immune status
d.  Reassure the patient because rubella is not a problem until after the 30th week
e.  Terminate the pregnancy

**105.** Mad cow disease has been highly publicized worldwide. Human infection starts with a change in cerebral function, usually diagnosed with a psychiatric disorder that ends in death after 4–5 years. This disease is caused by which of the following?

a.  A prion
b.  A virus
c.  A bacterium with a defective cell wall
d.  An autoimmune reaction
e.  *Rickettsia rickettsiae*

**106.** A traveler visited a geographic area where hepatitis A was endemic and did not remember to take gamma globulin for passive protection. Four weeks later, he experienced fever, nausea, and jaundice, with dark urine. HAV infection was suspected, but all the tests for HAV-IgG and HAV-IgM were nonreactive. Which of the following is the most likely cause of this infection?

a.  Hepatitis B surface antigen
b.  Hepatitis C
c.  Hepatitis D
d.  Hepatitis E
e.  Rotavirus

**107.** A 70-year-old nursing home patient refused the influenza vaccine and subsequently developed influenza. She died of acute pneumonia 1 week after contracting the flu. Which of the following is the most common cause of acute postinfluenzal pneumonia?

a.  *Escherichia coli*
b.  *Klebsiella pneumoniae*
c.  *Legionella pneumophilia*
d.  *Listeria monocytogenes*
e.  *Staphylococcus aureus*

**108.** A 5-year-old boy was sent home from kindergarten because his left eye was red with a watery, nonpurulent discharge. Several of his classmates recently had mild sore throat but no fever. Conjunctivitis lasted 1 week with complete recovery. Which of the following organisms was the most likely cause of his infection?

a.  Adenovirus
b.  Herpes simplex virus
c.  Staphylococcus aureus
d.  Chlamydiae trachomatis
e.  Hemophilus aegypticus

**109.** A husband and wife performed the yearly spring cleaning of their mountain cabin, located in the southwestern part of the United States. The wife presented to her physician 2 weeks later with fever, myalgia, headache, and nausea, followed by progressive pulmonary edema. Which of the following statements best describes the pathogen or disease progression in this patient?

a.  Hemolysis is common in infected patients
b.  Influenza-like symptoms are followed rapidly by acute respiratory failure
c.  It is acquired by inhalation of aerosols of the urine and feces of deer
d.  Transmission from human to human is common
e.  There is effective antiviral therapy available

**110.** Which of the following statements best applies to the oncogenes of DNA viruses?

a. They are early viral genes that perform essential viral functions
b. They are cell genes that are expressed during embryonic development
c. They encode a protein that has tyrosine kinase–like activity
d. They are virtually identical to the oncogenes of RNA tumor viruses
e. They are cell genes accidentally incorporated into the viral genome

**111.** Which of the following viruses may be a definitive human tumor virus?

a. Epstein-Barr virus (EBV)
b. Herpes simplex virus, type 2 (HSV-2)
c. HIV
d. Papillomavirus
e. Varicella-zoster virus (VZV)

**112.** Parvovirus infection, the cause of a mild exanthem in children, can also cause which of the following?

a. Aplastic crisis in chronic anemia
b. Epidemic acute respiratory disease
c. Gastroenteritis
d. Keratoconjunctivitis
e. Whooping cough-like disease

**113.** Within the first year of life, an infant exhibited severe hearing loss, ocular abnormalities, and apparent mental retardation. Standard peripheral blood smears demonstrated multinucleated cells with giant nuclei and intranuclear inclusions. Which of the following statements best describes the etiologic agent?

a. It can be transmitted across the placental barrier
b. While a common infection, CMV is almost always symptomatic
c. The CMV can be cultured from red blood cells of infected patients
d. Unlike other viral infections, CMV is not activated by immunosuppressive therapy
e. There is no specific therapy for CMV

**114.** An outbreak of acute viral gastroenteritis occurred in a child-care center, with several very young children exhibiting nausea, vomiting, and watery, nonbloody diarrhea. Which of the following statements characterizes routine human rotavirus infections?

a. They produce an infection that is seen primarily in adults
b. They produce cytopathic effects in many conventional tissue culture systems
c. They are lipid-containing RNA viruses possessing a double-shelled capsid
d. They can be sensitively and rapidly detected in stools by the ELISA technique
e. They have been implicated as a major etiologic agent of infantile respiratory disease

**115.** Subacute sclerosing panencephalitis (SSPE) is characterized by inflammatory lesions and begins with mild changes in personality, ending with dementia and death. Which of the following statements best describes the disease characteristics?

a. Demyelination is characteristic
b. It is a common event occurring in 1 of 300,000 cases of mumps
c. It is a late CNS manifestation of mumps
d. It is a progressive disease involving both white and gray matter
e. Viral DNA can be demonstrated in brain cells

**116.** The virus shown below contains double-stranded RNA within a double-walled capsid. Which of the following statements best describes this agent?

a. Early breast-feeding offers no protection to neonates against it
b. It is a major cause of neonatal diarrhea
c. It is readily cultured from the stool of infected persons
d. Maternal antibody does not appear to be protective
e. There are no related animal viruses

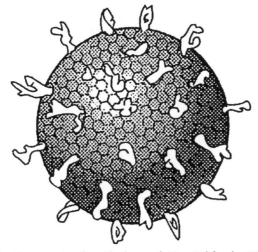

*(Reproduced, with permission, from Bhushan et al.* First Aid for the USMLE Step 1. A Student to Student Guide, *2006. New York, McGraw-Hill, 2006: 155.)*

**117.** Helical viruses containing negative sense linear RNA genomes and an outer lipid envelope are most commonly associated with which of the following diseases?

a. Croup
b. Fifth disease
c. Otitis media
d. Rubella
e. Tonsillitis

**118.** A transplant patient taking high levels of immunosuppressive medications becomes infected with EBV and develops a lymphoma. The dosage of immunosuppressive drugs given to the patient is decreased, and the tumor regresses. Which of the following properties of EBV infection is related to the patient's tumor development?

a. Immortalization of B cells
b. Increased white blood cell count
c. Presence of atypical lymphocytes
d. Production of heterophile antibodies

**119.** Reverse transcriptase is an enzyme found in retroviruses and hepadnaviruses. Which of the following is a function of the enzyme reverse transcriptase?

a. DNAse activity
b. DNA-dependent RNA polymerase activity
c. RNA-dependent DNA polymerase activity
d. RNA-dependent RNA polymerase activity
e. RNA isomerase activity

**120.** Several young adults camped in a wilderness area and received multiple mosquito bites. Ten days later, one had a sudden onset of headache, chills, and fever, and became stuporous 48 hours later. He was diagnosed with Saint Louis encephalitis (SLE) and recovered completely. Which of the following best describes SLE?

a. It is transmitted to humans by the bite of an infected tick
b. It is caused by a togavirus
c. It is the major arboviral cause of central nervous system infection in the United States
d. It may present initially with symptoms similar to influenza
e. Laboratory diagnosis is routinely made by cultural methods

**121.** There is considerable overlap of signs and symptoms seen in congenital and perinatal infections. In a neonate with classic symptoms of congenital CMV infection, which of the following tests would be most useful in establishing a diagnosis?

a.  CMV IgG titer on neonate's serum at birth
b.  CMV IgG titer on mother's serum at birth of infant
c.  CMV IgM titer on neonate's serum at birth and at 1 month of age
d.  Culture of mother's urine
e.  Total IgM on neonate's serum at birth

**122.** IFNs are host-coded proteins that are cytokines and are produced within hours of microbial infection. IFN's then modulate humoral and cellular immunity. Which of the following stimulates IFN production in patients and cells in tissue culture?

a.  Botulinum toxin
b.  Chlamydiae
c.  Gram-positive bacteria
d.  Synthetic polypeptides
e.  Viruses

**123.** A 35-year-old man presents with symptoms of jaundice, right upper quadrant pain, and vomiting. His ALT is elevated. He is diagnosed with HAV infection after eating at a restaurant where others were also infected. Which of the following should be done to protect his family members?

a.  A series of three vaccinations at 0, 1, and 6 months
b.  Administer alpha interferon
c.  Quarantine household contacts and observe
d.  No treatment is necessary
e.  One dose of gamma globulin administered intramuscularly

**124.** A 17-year-old girl presents with cervical lymphadenopathy, fever, and pharyngitis. Which of the following is the most rapid and clinically useful test to make a diagnosis?

a.  Antibody to Epstein-Barr nuclear antigen (EBNA)
b.  C-reactive protein (CRP)
c.  Culture
d.  IgG antibody to viral core antigen (VCA)
e.  IgM antibody to VCA

**125.** A latent infection is usually manifested by persistence of viral genomes, expression of no or a few viral genes, and survival of the infected cells. Reactivation may occur sporadically or not at all, usually dependent upon immune competence. Which of the following viruses would be most likely to establish a latent infection?

a. Adenovirus
b. Coxsackievirus group B
c. Influenza virus
d. Measles virus
e. Poliovirus

**126.** On November 6, a patient had the onset of an illness characterized by fever, chills, headache, cough, and chest pain. The illness lasted 1 week. On December 5, she had another illness very similar to the first, which lasted 6 days. She had no flu immunization during this period. Her hemagglutination inhibition (HI) antibody titer to swine flu virus was as follows:

November 6      10
November 30     10
December 20     160
(There was no laboratory error)

Which of the following is the best conclusion from these data?

a. The patient was ill with swine flu on November 6
b. The patient was ill with swine flu later, and the November 6 illness was due to another pathogen
c. The patient was ill with swine flu on December 20
d. It is impossible to relate either illness with the specific virus

**127.** Atypical lymphocytosis is most likely to be found in which one of the following diseases?

a. Encephalitis caused by herpes simplex virus (HSV)
b. Chronic hepatitis C
c. Mononucleosis induced by Epstein-Barr virus
d. Parvovirus infection
e. Rotavirus gastroenteritis

**128.** A tourist who recently returned from a Caribbean cruise suddenly develops arthralgia, a maculopapular rash, and lymphadenopathy with back and bone pain. Which of the following is the most likely diagnosis?

a. Dengue fever
b. Hepatitis
c. HIV infection
d. Infectious mononucleosis
e. Saint Louis encephalitis

**129.** A 30-year-old female with a recent history of serious illness requiring surgery developed fever, nausea, and jaundice. Her condition continued as a clinically mild disease, with AST=552, ALT=712, and the HBV panel was negative. Which one of the following statements best characterizes the illness?

a. Blood products are not tested for antibody to HCV
b. Few cases progress to chronic liver disease
c. HBV but not HCV infections occur in IV drug abusers
d. HCV is a DNA virus
e. HCV is the most common cause of posttransfusion hepatitis

**130.** Which of the following markers is usually the first viral marker detected after hepatitis B infection?

a. HBcAg
b. HBeAg
c. HBsAg
d. HBeAb
e. Anti–HBc

**131.** Which of the following may be the only detectable serological marker during the early convalescent phase of HBV infection (window phase)?

a. HBcAg
b. HBeAg
c. HBsAg
d. HBeAb
e. Anti–HBc

**132.** Which of the following markers is closely associated with HBV infectivity and DNA polymerase activity?

a. HBcAg
b. HBeAg
c. HBsAg
d. HBeAb
e. Anti–HBc

**133.** Which of the following is found within the nuclei of infected hepatocytes and not usually in the peripheral circulation?

a. HBcAg
b. HBeAg
c. HBsAg
d. HBeAb
e. Anti–HBc

**134.** An infant was born and presented with intrauterine growth retardation, jaundice, hepatosplenomegaly, microcephaly, and retinitis. Which one of the following viruses most likely caused these congenital malformations?

a. Cytomegalovirus
b. Mumps
c. HIV
d. Respiratory syncytial virus
e. Rubeola

**135.** A 20-year-old male experienced a paramyxovirus infection and developed a high fever at the end of the first week of illness. This was accompanied by swelling, tenderness, and severe pain in the testes that lasted 5 days. This infection was a manifestation of which of the following viruses?

a. Cytomegalovirus
b. Mumps
c. Rabies
d. Respiratory syncytial virus
e. Rubeola

**136.** Antigenic drift and antigenic shift refer to influenza viruses. Which of the following statements describes events that could lead to a new influenza epidemic?

a. Antigenic drift represents the sudden appearance of new subtypes of HA and/or NA
b. Antigenic drift represents a gradual change in the HA and/or NA antigens
c. Antigenic shift represents the sudden appearance of new subtypes of HA and/or NA
d. Antigenic shift represents a gradual change in HA and/or NA antigens
e. Antigenic shift results in the inactivation of interferons

**137.** Which of the following viruses may enter the central nervous system (CNS) at neuromuscular junctions or directly into the CNS without replication, resulting in a fatal encephalitis, and may be prevented by a vaccine?

a. Cytomegalovirus
b. Mumps
c. Rabies
d. Respiratory syncytial virus
e. Rhinovirus

**138.** Although vaccination with live, attenuated, or killed viral vaccines has been the most effective way of controlling viral disease in the population, common colds remain widespread because of the multiple serotypes identified. Which of the following viruses represents this problem ?

a. CMV
b. Mumps
c. Rabies
d. Respiratory syncytial virus
e. Rhinovirus

**139.** HAV contains RNA and principally infects children in lower socioeconomic conditions, although outbreaks in commercial eating establishments may involve all age groups. Acute, but not chronic, infections occur. Which of the following is available and effective for HAV control?

a. Acyclovir
b. Inactivated virus vaccine
c. Killed virus vaccine
d. Live virus vaccine
e. Recombinant viral vaccine

**140.** Uncomplicated influenza appears abruptly, with chills, headache, and dry cough, followed by high fever, muscle aches and malaise, and anorexia, usually lasting 3–5 days. All age groups may be affected during the yearly flu season. In order to prevent infections and frequent complications, individuals should be vaccinated annually with which of the following vaccines?

a. Immune serum globulin
b. Inactivated/killed virus vaccine
c. Purified HA/NA preparations
d. Live virus vaccine
e. Recombinant viral vaccine

**141.** Rubeola is an acute, highly infectious disease, characterized by fever, respiratory symptoms, and a maculopapular rash. Which of the following best characterizes the vaccine that has dramatically reduced the incidence of this disease in the United States?

a. Bacterin
b. Inactivated virus vaccine
c. Killed virus vaccine
d. Live virus vaccine
e. Recombinant viral vaccine

**142.** HSV incidence remains high in the population, although control measures are available. Which of the following is the treatment of choice for HSV infection?

a. Acyclovir
b. Azythromycin
c. Herpes immune globulin
d. Killed virus vaccine
e. Recombinant viral vaccine

**143.** Viral vaccines continue to be the most effective mechanism of controlling disease in the population, even though chemotherapy and IFNs are available. Which of the following best describes the presently available vaccine for hepatitis B?

a. Inactivated virus vaccine
b. Killed virus vaccine
c. Live virus vaccine
d. Recombinant viral vaccine
e. Synthetic peptide vaccine

**144.** Two weeks after contact with an individual with an acute disease presentation, a 12-year-old girl has fever and malaise, followed by a rash composed of crops of vesicles which lasts 5 days. This common childhood disease is caused by which of the following viruses?

a. Adenovirus
b. Cytomegalovirus
c. Papillomavirus
d. Rubeola
e. Varicella virus

**145.** A new military recruit presents with acute conjunctivitis. Which of the following agents is the most likely cause?

a. Adenovirus
b. Cytomegalovirus
c. Papillomavirus
d. Rotavirus
e. Varicella virus

**146.** Small icosahedral DNA viruses are highly tropic for epithelial cells of the skin and mucus membranes. Which of the following can cause cosmetically unsightly lesions or lead to a form of cancer?

a. Adenovirus
b. Cytomegalovirus
c. Papillomavirus
d. Rotavirus
e. Varicella virus

**147.** Which of the following is a medium-sized virus capable of experiencing genetic reassortment, which recently had an approved vaccine recalled because of bowel blockage complications?

a. Adenovirus
b. Cytomegalovirus
c. Papillomavirus
d. Rotavirus
e. Varicella virus

**148.** A child has mononucleosis-like symptoms, yet the tests for mononucleosis and the EBV titers are negative. Which of the following is a cause of heterophile-negative mononucleosis?

a. Adenovirus
b. Coxsackievirus
c. Cytomegalovirus
d. Herpes simplex virus
e. Varicella-zoster virus

**149.** Malaise and fatigue with increased "atypical" lymphocytes and a reactive heterophil antibody test are most commonly caused by which of the following?

a. *Borrelia burgdorferi*
b. Epstein-Barr virus
c. Parvovirus
d. Rubella virus
e. *Toxoplasma*

**150.** A patient has complement fixation antibody titers against measles virus as follows: acute = 40, convalescent = 80. Which of the following is the correct conclusion concerning this patient?

a. The patient has a recurrent, acute infection
b. Infection occurred sometime in the past
c. The antibodies could only have been made due to vaccination
d. The patient would be incompletely immune to measles due to lack of CMI immunity
e. An immediate booster shot would be necessary to enhance the patient's protection against measles

**151.** A tumor of the jaw in African children may be characterized by elevated "early antigen" tests with a restricted pattern of fluorescence. This disease is caused by which of the following?

a. *Borrelia burgdorferi*
b. Cytomegalovirus
c. Epstein-Barr virus
d. Herpes simplex virus
e. Lymphogranuloma venereum

**152.** Which of the following viruses may be detected by the polymerase chain reaction (PCR) in a variety of cells of patients with nasopharyngeal carcinoma?

a. Epstein-Barr virus
b. Measles
c. Mumps
d. Parvovirus
e. Rubella

**153.** A 2-day-old newborn with a mononucleosis-like syndrome has microcephaly, cataracts, and "owl eye" cytopathic effects in biopsy tissue cells. Which of the following viruses is the most likely cause of this infection?

a. Cytomegalovirus
b. Epstein-Barr virus
c. HHV-6
d. Norwalk virus
e. Parvovirus

**154.** Which of the following specimens is best for detection of human papillomavirus (HPV)?

a. Blood
b. Cervical tissue
c. Skin
d. Synovial fluid

**155.** Which of the following specimens is best for detection of cytomegalovirus (CMV)?

a. Blood
b. Cerebrospinal fluid
c. Cervical tissue
d. Skin
e. Synovial fluid

**156.** Which of the following specimens is best for detection of enterovirus?

a. Blood
b. Cerebrospinal fluid
c. Cervical tissue
d. Skin
e. Synovial fluid

**157.** Which of the following specimens is best for detection of varicella-zoster virus (VZV)?

a. Blood
b. Cerebrospinal fluid
c. Cervical tissue
d. Skin
e. Synovial fluid

**158.** Which of the following specimens is best for detection of adenovirus 40/41?

a. Blood
b. Cerebrospinal fluid
c. Cervical tissue
d. Stool
e. Synovial fluid

**159.** Twenty-five days following consumption of shellfish, a 35-year-old man presents with acute jaundice and liver function abnormalities. Which of the following is the most likely cause of his infection?

a. Adenovirus 40/41
b. Astrovirus
c. Hepatitis A virus
d. Norwalk virus
e. Rotavirus

**160.** Which of the following viruses causes only gastroenteritis and is the *second* most common cause of pediatric gastroenteritis?

a. Adenovirus 40/41
b. Astrovirus
c. Hepatitis A virus
d. Norwalk virus
e. Rotavirus

**161.** Which of the following is difficult to grow in cell culture but can be detected easily by immunologic methods (ELISA), and is the most common cause of pediatric gastroenteritis?

a. Adenovirus 40/41
b. Astrovirus
c. Hepatitis A virus
d. Norwalk virus
e. Rotavirus

**162.** Which of the following may be detected by ELISA methods or electron microscopy and is a common cause of epidemic gastroenteritis, particularly aboard cruise ships and in summer camps?

a. Adenovirus 40/41
b. Astrovirus
c. Hepatitis A virus
d. Norwalk virus
e. Rotavirus

**163.** Unlike other similar viruses, this agent appears to account for 5–15% of the gastroenteritis in young children. Which of the following etiologic agents causes these infections and is difficult to isolate in the diagnostic laboratory?

a. Adenovirus 40/41
b. Astrovirus
c. Hepatitis A virus
d. Norwalk virus
e. Rotavirus

**164.** Rubella is a common cause of examthems in children and is best described by which of the following statements?

a.  Incubation time is approximately 3–4 weeks
b.  Infections routinely fail to generate an immune response
c.  It can be diagnosed by the presence of Koplik's spots
d.  Rubeola and rubella are caused by the same virus
e.  Specific antibody in the serum does prevent disease

**165.** Which of the following viruses belongs to the family of flaviviruses, its reservoir is strictly human, and transmission is bloodborne, so the blood supply is routinely screened for it?

a.  Hepatitis A
b.  Hepatitis B
c.  Hepatitis C
d.  Hepatitis D
e.  Hepatitis E

**166.** Vaccination for this hepatic disease is with viral surface antigen and usually provides immunity to which of the following viruses?

a.  Hepatitis A
b.  Hepatitis B
c.  Hepatitis C
d.  Hepatitis D
e.  Hepatitis E

**167.** This hepatitis virus is a calicivirus. The reservoir is in pigs, and humans acquire it via the fecal-oral route. Which of the following is the virus?

a.  Hepatitis A
b.  Hepatitis B
c.  Hepatitis C
d.  Hepatitis D
e.  Hepatitis E

**168.** This hepatitis virus is a defective virus in that it cannot replicate independently without the presence of hepatitis B virus. Which of the following is the virus?

a.  Hepatitis A
b.  Hepatitis B
c.  Hepatitis C
d.  Hepatitis D
e.  Hepatitis E

**169.** Viruses have various ways of entering the human body and producing disease. Which of the following descriptions accurately describes the route and mechanism for the virus indicated?

a.  Coronaviruses enter the gastrointestinal tract through the mouth and move into the stomach, where they proliferate within mucosal cells to produce peptic ulcers
b.  Enteroviruses enter through the mouth, replicate in the pharynx and bowel, and move via the blood to distant target organs (central nervous system)
c.  HIV is directly injected into the bloodstream by insects requiring blood for egg development
d.  Influenza viruses enter through the respiratory tract, replicate within lymphocytes in the lung, and move via the lymphatic vessels to joints and the CNS to produce muscle aches, stiff joints, and fever
e.  Mumps virus enters through abraded skin in the genital area and moves into the testicles of males to produce swelling and sterility

**170.** A flavivirus recently appeared in the United States with birds as the primary hosts. The virus produces viremia in humans and possible fatal encephalitis in older patients. Which of the following is this virus?

a.  Human papillomavirus
b.  *Polyomavirus*
c.  Subacute sclerosing panencephalitis (SSPE) virus
d.  Tick-borne encephalitis virus
e.  West Nile virus

**171.** Which of the following viruses causes progressive multifocal leukoencephalopathy (PML), a disease causing demyelination in the CNS in immunocompromized individuals?

a.  Human papillomavirus
b.  *Polyomavirus*
c.  Subacute sclerosing panencephalitis (SSPE) virus
d.  Tick-borne encephalitis virus
e.  West Nile virus

**172.** An irritable 18-month-old toddler with fever and blister-like ulcerations on mucous membranes of the oral cavity refuses to eat. The symptoms worsen and then slowly resolve over a period of 2 weeks. Assuming that the etiological agent was HSV type 1, which of the following statements is true?

a.  Antivirals do not provide any benefit
b.  The virus remains latent in the trigeminal ganglia
c.  Recurrence is likely to result in a generalized rash
d.  Polyclonal B cell activation is a prominent feature
e.  The child is at high risk for developing cancer later in life

**173.** A sexually active 17-year-old man presents to the local free clinic to check some small papules that appeard on his penis. The papules are small, white lesions with a central depression. There is no discharge or pain on urination. What group listed below does this etiologic agent belong to?

a.  Adenoviridae
b.  Arenaviridae
c.  Papovaviridae
d.  Parvoviridae
e.  Poxviridae

**174.** A fifth-grade student with a maculopapular rash attended class and was sent home at noontime. Two weeks later, three classmates developed fever, coughing, running nose, and white ulcerations on the buccal mucosa before developing a similar rash. Which of the following viruses caused these infections?

a.  Adenovirus
b.  Influenza virus
c.  Measles virus
d.  Parainfluenza virus
e.  Respiratory syncytial virus

**175.** Which of the following viruses is the leading cause of bronchiolitis and community-acquired pneumonia in infants?

a.  Adenovirus
b.  Influenza virus
c.  Measles virus
d.  Parainfluenza virus
e.  Respiratory syncytial virus

**176.** Which of the following viral infections is localized, lacking a viremic stage, and chiefly dependent on secretory IgA for viral neutralization?

a.  Coronavirus
b.  Measles virus
c.  Mumps virus
d.  Respiratory syncytial virus
e.  Variola major

**177.** Which of the following viruses is a double-stranded DNA virus responsible for 15% of pediatric respiratory infections and 10–15% of acute diarrhea in children?

a.  Adenovirus
b.  Influenza virus
c.  Measles virus
d.  Parainfluenza virus
e.  Respiratory syncytial virus

# Virology

## Answers

**64. The answer is d.** (*Murray—2003, pp 1271–1272. Ryan, pp 614–615.*) HIV RT PCR, a nucleic acid amplification test for HIV RNA, has recently been shown to be the most valuable test for (a) monitoring a patient's progress during triple drug therapy and (b) determining the chances of progression to AIDS. A viral load of 100,000–750,000 copies per milliliter significantly increases the chance of progression to AIDS within 5 years. The amount of HIV in the blood (viral load) is of significant prognostic value. The steady-state level of virus (virus replication vs viral killing) reflects the number of infected cells and the average burst size. Plasma HIV quantitative RNA levels can be determined by the RT PCR and appears to be the best predictor of long-term clinical outcome. CD4 counts appear to be the best predictor of short-term risk of developing an opportunistic infection. Effectiveness of antiretroviral drug therapy is most often assessed by RT PCR assays. The other tests listed do not accurately predict progression to AIDS. The following figure shows the basic structure of HIV, including the enzyme reverse transcriptase.

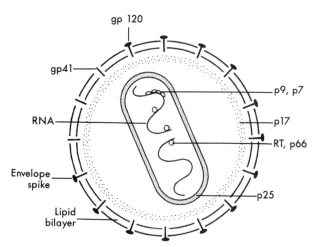

The location of the envelope glycoproteins (gp 120 and gp 124) is shown, as are the major viral core proteins (p 25, p 17, p 9, and p 7). The core protein, p 17, is found outside the viral nucleoid and forms the matrix of the virion. RT indicates reverse transcriptase.

**65. The answer is b.** (*Murray—2005, pp 574–576. Ryan, pp 522–523.*) Parvovirus B19 is the causative agent of erythema infectiosum (fifth disease). It is associated with transient aplastic crisis in persons with hereditary hemolytic anemia. In adults, it is also associated with polyarthralgia (and fetal loss in pregnant women). Serology detects specific IgM antibody to Parvovirus.

**66. The answer is c.** (*Gilligan, pp 47–50. Murray—2005, pp 545–547. Ryan, p 558.*) The initial infection by HSV is often inapparent and occurs through a break in the skin or mucous membranes, such as in the eye, throat, or genitals. Latent infection often persists at the initial site despite high antibody titers. Recurrent disease can be triggered by temperature change, emotional distress, and hormonal factors. Type 1 HSV is usually, but not exclusively, associated with ocular and oral lesions; type 2 is usually, but not exclusively, associated with genital and anal lesions. Type 2 infection is more common. In addition to mucocutaneous infections, the CNS and occasionally visceral organs can be involved.

**67–69. The answers are 67-d, 68-e, 69-d.** (*Levinson, pp 291, 320, 313–321. Murray—2005, pp 670–671. Ryan, pp 615–616.*) The advent of triple therapy, or a therapeutic "cocktail," has had a marked effect on AIDS patients. The combination of drugs works together as reverse transcriptive inhibitors and a protease inhibitor. Patients improve rapidly, their CD4 lymphocyte counts increase, and their HIV viral loads are drastically reduced, often to less than 50 copies per milliliter. On the other hand, an untreated HIV-positive patient with a low CD4 and a high viral load (a) is at increased risk of opportunistic infection and (b) has a much greater chance of developing AIDS than if the viral load was less than 10,000. The patient is infectious and his HIV antibody screening test will be positive. The high viral load, however, is not a predictor of response to therapy. Many patients with high viral loads do very well on triple therapy, although resistance to one or more of the agents may subsequently occur. A low CD4 count does not predict progression to AIDS but does indicate increased chance of opportunistic infection such as those listed. Kaposi sarcoma, which has been linked to herpesvirus type 8, pneumocystis, and mycobacterial disease are three of the most prevalent opportunistic infections. While HIV-positive patients contract pneumococcal pneumonia, they are probably at no more risk than the general population, as protection against pneumococcal disease is linked to the presence of anticapsular antibody.

**70. The answer is e.** (*Murray—2005, pp 553–558. Ryan, pp 571–573.*) All of Koch's postulates have been verified for the relationship between infectious mononucleosis and EBV, a herpesvirus. However, the relationship between this virus and Burkitt's lymphoma, sarcoid, and systemic lupus erythematosus (SLE) is less clear. Infectious mononucleosis is most common in young adults (14–18 years of age) and is very rare in young children. There is no specific treatment. Heterophil antibody titer is helpful in diagnosis, but is not expressed as a function of clinical recovery.

**71. The answer is b.** (*Brooks, pp 615–616. Levinson, pp 320. Murray—2005, pp 670–671. Ryan, pp 614–615.*) The standard screening test for HIV antibody detection is the ELISA. It is well standardized and available in kit format for relative ease of use in laboratories. As a screening test, however, some false-positive and false-negative results may occasionally be obtained. The standard practice, therefore, is to always perform a second ELISA test before reporting any test result. In fact, before any final report in HIV diagnosis is sent out, a confirming test (Western blot test, in most cases) will need to be performed. HIV culture is not routinely done. No evidence of P. carinii was noted in the history. Until confirmed, no AZT use is justified and, certainly, no suggestion of AIDS development would be made on the basis of screening test results.

**72. The answer is b.** (*Murray—2005, pp 637–638. Ryan, pp 587–593.*) Arboviruses (arthropod-borne viruses) may or may not be surrounded by a lipid envelope, although most are inactivated by lipid solvents such as ether and may contain either double-stranded or single-stranded RNA. Physicochemical studies have demonstrated a great heterogeneity among these viruses. Arboviruses cause disease in vertebrates; in humans, encephalitis is a frequent arbovirus illness. Most human infections with arbovirus, however, are asymptomatic.

**73. The answer is d.** (*Levinson, pp 221–222. Murray—2005, pp 144–146. Ryan, p 104.*) IFN is a protein produced by cells in response to a viral infection or certain other agents. Entering uninfected cells, IFN causes production of a second protein (AVP-antiviral protein) that alters protein synthesis. As a result of inhibition of either translation or transcription, new viruses are not assembled following infection of IFN-protected cells.

**74. The answer is b.** *(Brooks, pp 570–574. Murray—2005, pp 591–594. Ryan, p 511.)* Coronaviruses, discovered in 1965, are thought to be a major agent of the common cold, especially in older children and adults. The virion is known to contain RNA, but other elements of its structure are unclear. At 34°C, viral multiplication is profuse; however, infectivity is greatly reduced at higher temperatures or following extended incubation. Rhinoviruses (picornaviruses) are the other major cause of common cold. There is no common connection between the SARS agent and those causing colds. Coronaviruses may also cause gastroenteritis in humans, although these agents have not been isolated.

**75. The answer is b.** *(Levinson, pp 291–292. Murray—2005, pp 687–689. Ryan, pp 550–551.)* The delta agent was first described in 1977 and has recently been shown to be a defective RNA virus that requires HBsAg for replication. It is found most often in persons who have multiple parenteral exposures—for example, intravenous (IV) drug abusers, hemophiliacs, and multiply transfused patients.

**76. The answer is c.** *(Brooks, p 531, 560. Murray—2005, pp 505, 509, 607. Ryan, pp 209–210.)* As an IV agent, ribavirin is effective against Lassa fever in the first week of onset of the disease. It may also be administered as an aerosol that is quite useful in infants with RSV. Unlike amantadine, which is efficacious only with influenza A, ribavirin has activity against both influenza A and influenza B if administered by aerosol in the first 24 hours of onset.

**77. The answer is d.** *(Brooks, pp 497–499. Murray—2005, pp 585–586. Ryan, pp 537–539.)* Echoviruses were discovered accidentally during studies on poliomyelitis. They were named echoviruses because, at the time, they had not been linked to human disease and thus were considered "orphans." Echoviruses now are known to infect the intestinal tract of humans; they also can cause aseptic meningitis, febrile illnesses, and the common cold. Echoviruses range in size from 24–30 nm in diameter and contain a core of RNA.

**78. The answer is d.** *(Ryan, pp 561–562. Brooks, pp 433–438. Murray—2005, pp 546–549.)* HSV meningitis or encephalitis is difficult to diagnose by laboratory tests, as there is a low titer of virus present in the CSF. Neonatal

HSV infects the child during the birth process. While culture, Tzanck smear, and even antibody tests may be useful in adults, particularly those with HSV-rich lesions, they are not useful for CSF testing. Only PCR is sensitive enough to detect HSV DNA in the CSF. Once diagnosed rapidly, HSV encephalitis or meningitis can be treated with acyclovir.

**79. The answer is b.** (*Brooks, p 495–497. Levinson, p 279. Murray—2005, pp 585–586.*) Enterovirus and coxsackievirus A can be recovered from conjunctival scrapings of patients with AHC during the first 3 days of illness. Isolation rates are somewhat higher for enterovirus than for coxsackievirus. Less than 5% of throat swab or fecal specimens have been positive for either virus. Echovirus 70 is the chief cause of this disease.

**80. The answer is c.** (*Brooks, pp 560–562. Levinson, pp 266–267. Murray—2005, pp 605–607. Ryan, pp 514–515.*) Much of the public's understanding of mumps is based on suppositions that are without any scientific basis. For example, natural mumps infection confers immunity after a single infection, even if the infection was a unilateral, not a bilateral, parotitis. Also, sterility from mumps orchitis is not ensured; only 20% of males older than 13 years of age develop orchitis. The majority of patients with mumps do not develop systemic manifestations. In fact, some do not develop parotitis. Last, the virus is maintained exclusively in human populations; canine reservoirs are not known. The mumps vaccine is a live attenuated virus vaccine derived from chick-embryo tissue culture.

**81. The answer is e.** (*Brooks, pp 438–442. Levinson, pp 248–249. Murray—2005, pp 550–553. Ryan, pp 563–565.*) This is a classic description for a reactivation of varicella-zoster viral latent infection. Many initial infections with VZV are subclinical and result in latent infections in sensory ganglion nerve tissue. Varicella (chickenpox) is mild and highly contagious in children. Zoster (shingles) is a sporadic, incapacitating illness seen in adults. Treatment may include acyclovir or famciclovir. Herpes B virus infections occur primarily in monkeys. HSV primary infections are most often subclinical and occur primarily in children. EBV (infectious mononucleosis) persists in latent infections in B lymphocytes.

**82. The answer is c.** (*Brooks, pp 562–566. Levinson, pp 264–266. Murray—2005, pp 598–603. Ryan, pp 517–518.*) Koplik's spots are pathognomonic for measles. The measles virus is a paramyxovirus. In industrialized countries, vaccination has reduced the importance of this childhood infection (although U.S. incidence increased in 1989 and 1990). In developing countries, however, measles is a major killer of young children. In America, most states now require proof of immunity before school enrollment, and this has reduced the incidence of disease.

**83. The answer is e.** *(Brooks, pp 599–601. Levinson, pp 256–257. Murray—2005, pp 523–524. Ryan, p 619.)* HPV is the cause of genital warts. It is one of the most pervasive of all the sexually transmitted diseases. There is no specific cure or vaccine. There are multiple serotypes of papillomavirus, and some serotypes are linked to cervical cancer. New techniques for molecular diagnosis of HPV show promise for rapid and sensitive detection and perhaps more aggressive treatment. HSV-II was originally thought to be etiologically involved, but is now not considered so. HSV-II evidence came primarily from serological data.

**84. The answer is c.** *(Brooks, pp 554–558. Levinson, p 268. Murray—2005, pp 603–604. Ryan, pp 506–507.)* Parainfluenza viruses are important causes of respiratory diseases in infants and young children. The spectrum of disease caused by these viruses ranges from a mild febrile cold to croup, bronchiolitis, and pneumonia. Parainfluenza viruses contain RNA in a nucleocapsid encased within an envelope derived from the host cell membrane. Infected mammalian cell culture will hemabsorb red blood cells owing to viral hemagglutinin on the surface of the cell.

**85. The answer is a.** *(Brooks, p 470. Levinson, p 292. Murray—2005, pp 677, 689.)* Hepatitis E is a newly recognized single-stranded RNA virus in the calicivirus family. Epidemics have been observed in Asia, Africa, India, and Mexico. Like HAV, it is enterically transmitted, but there is no vaccine available nor is there a routine detection test. Chronic liver disease does not occur, and because it is not bloodborne, it is of no threat to the blood supply.

**86. The answer is e.** *(Brooks, p 736.)* Aseptic meningitis is characterized by a pleocytosis of mononuclear cells in the CSF; polymorphonuclear cells predominate during the first 24 hours, but a shift to lymphocytes occurs thereafter. The CSF of affected persons is free of culturable bacteria and contains normal glucose and slightly elevated protein levels. Peripheral white blood cell counts usually are normal. Although viruses are the most common cause of aseptic meningitis, spirochetes, chlamydiae, and other microorganisms also can produce the disease.

CSF findings

Bacterial: pressure ↑, polys ↑, proteins ↑, glucose ↓.

Viral: pressure normal / ↑, lymphs ↑, proteins normal, glucose normal.

TB/fungal: pressure ↑, lymphs ↑, proteins ↑, glucose ↓.

**87. The answer is c.** *(Brooks, pp 466–469.)* Although HBcIgM is present in acute stages, in a chronic HBV carrier, there would be no HB core IgM antibody, whereas it would be present in a new HBV infection. The HBe antigen could be present in either an HBV carrier or in acute infection. HBsAg would be present in either a new infection or in the carrier state, while HBsAb would not be present in either case.

**88. The answer is e.** *(Brooks, pp 466–469. Levinson, pp 283–291. Murray— 2005, pp 678–685. Ryan, p 549.)* In a small number of patients with acute hepatitis B infection, HBsAg can never be detected. In others, HBsAg becomes negative before the onset of the disease or before the end of the clinical illness. In such patients with acute hepatitis, hepatitis B virus infection may be established only by the presence of anti–hepatitis B core IgM (anti–HBc IgM), a rising titer of anti–HBc, or the subsequent appearance of anti–HBsAg.

HBsAg positive, anti–HBs and anti–HBc negative would identify an early acute HBV infection. HBsAg and anti–HBc positive could indicate an acute or chronic HBV infection. IgM anti–HBc could differentiate between these conditions. HBsAg negative and anti–HBs positive tests indicate immunity due to natural infection or vaccination. Hepatitis symptoms and negative HBsAg, anti–HBs and anti–HBc test would indicate another infectious agent, toxic injury to the liver or possible disease of the biliary tract.

## INTERPRETATION OF HBV SEROLOGIC MARKERS IN PATIENTS WITH HEPATITIS*

| Assay Results | | | |
|---|---|---|---|
| **HBsAg** | **Anti-HBs** | **Anti-HBc** | **Interpretation** |
| Positive | Negative | Negative | Early acute HBV infection. Confirmation is required to exclude nonspecific reactivity. |
| Positive | (±) | Positive | HBV infection, either acute or chronic. Differentiate with IgM anti–HBc. Determine level of replicative activity (infectivity) with HBeAg or HBV DNA. |
| Negative | Positive | Positive | Indicates previous HBV infection and immunity to hepatitis B. |
| Negative | Negative | Positive | Possibilities include: HBV infection in remote past; "low-level" HBV carrier; "window" between disappearance of HBsAg and appearance of anti–HBs; or false-positive or nonspecific reaction. Investigate with IgM anti–HBc, challenge with HBsAg vaccine, or both. When present, anti–HBe helps validate the anti–HBc reactivity. |
| Negative | Negative | Negative | Another infectious agent, toxic injury to liver, disorder of immunity, hereditary disease of the liver, or disease of the biliary tract. |
| Negative | Positive | Negative | Vaccine-type response. |

*Modified and reproduced, with permission, from Hollinger FB. Hepatitis B virus. In: Fields BN et al (ed). Fields Virology, 3e. Lippincott-Raven, 1996.*

**89. The answer is d.** *(Brooks, pp 514–519. Levinson, pp 294–295.)* Eastern equine encephalitis (EEE) is a severe disease usually seen in the summer months when *Aedes* mosquitoes are prevalent. In 1996 and 1997, there were several outbreaks in the northeastern United States. Control of EEE is a function of mosquito eradication. Horses and humans are accidental hosts. If the patient survives, the CNS sequelae are usually severe. While draining of swamps helps, other measures to eliminate mosquitoes, such as spraying, are the most effective.

**90. The answer is c.** *(Brooks, pp 499–501. Levinson, p 275. Murray—2005, pp 588–589.)* Rhinovirus is a major cause of the common cold. The primary mode of transmission is the contact of contaminated hands, fingers, or fomites (fomites are objects such as clothing or utensils that can harbor or transmit a disease) with the conjunctiva or nasal epithelium. While several studies have shown no evidence of aerosol transmission, a study by Dick and associates in 1986 did show aerosol transmission can occur. This is not, however, the main mode of transmission.

**91. The answer is c.** *(Brooks, pp 562–566. Levinson, pp 262–264, 269–270. Murray—2005, pp 598–603. Ryan, pp 519–520.)* Measles (rubeola) caused by a paramyxovirus is an acute, highly infectious disease characterized by a maculopapular rash. German measles (rubella—a togavirus) is an acute, febrile illness characterized by a rash as well as suboccipital lymphadenopathy. Incubation time for measles is 9 full days after exposure. Onset is abrupt and symptoms mostly catarrhal. Koplik's spots, pale, bluish-white spots in red areolas, can frequently be observed on the mucous membranes of the mouth and are pathognomonic for measles.

**92. The answer is e.** *(Brooks, pp 575–581. Levinson, pp 271–272. Murray—2005, pp 619–623. Ryan, p 599.)* The definitive diagnosis of rabies in humans is based on the finding of Negri bodies, which are cytoplasmic inclusions in the nerve cells of the spinal cord and brain, especially in the hippocampus. Negri bodies are eosinophilic and generally spherical in shape; several may appear in a given cell. Negri bodies, although pathognomonic for rabies, are not found in all cases of the disease. In addition to CNS specimens, skin from the neck and at the hairline may be collected for microscopic examination.

**93. The answer is d.** *(Brooks, pp 582–584. Levinson, pp 189–190, 308–312. Murray—2005, pp 691–694. Ryan, pp 625–627.)* Kuru and CJD are similar but not identical diseases with very different epidemiology. Kuru is prevalent among certain tribes in New Guinea who practiced ritual cannibalism by eating the brains of the departed. CJD is found worldwide and has been transmitted by corneal transplants and in pituitary hormone preparations.

There is some association between CJD and mad cow disease in England. Prions are unconventional self-replicating proteins, sometimes called *amyloid*. It is now thought that CJD, kuru, and animal diseases such as scrapie, visna, and bovine spongiform encephalopathy (mad cow disease) are caused by prions.

**94. The answer is b.** (*Brooks, pp 456–461. Levinson, pp 252–253.*) Routine vaccination of infants and children for smallpox has been discontinued in the United States, both because the risk of contracting the disease is so low and because the complications of smallpox vaccination, including generalized vaccinia eruption, postvaccinal encephalitis, and fetal vaccinia, are significant. Owing to the extremely effective eradication of smallpox worldwide by the World Health Organization, U.S. citizens traveling abroad no longer require vaccination. Pregnancy, immune deficiencies, and eczema and other chronic dermatitides are contraindications to smallpox vaccination. Recent concerns about a possible terrorist attack involving smallpox have resulted in recommendations for using vaccinia vaccine on a limited scale, probably starting with health care workers.

**95. The answer is e.** (*Brooks, pp 575–581. Levinson, pp 271–272. Murray— 2005, pp 619–623. Ryan pp 597–600.*) Rabies is caused by a rhabdovirus (contains negative sense RNA, helical structure). The virus has a wide host of warm-blooded animals, including humans. The virus is widely distributed in the infected animals, with high levels in saliva. Street viruses (freshly isolated strains) have long incubation periods, leading to eventual viral infection of the CNS. Essentially, all organs are infected, giving rise to the described symptoms. Fixed (mutant) virus strains do not grow in neural tissue. Because of the long incubation period (weeks), active treatment (inactivated vaccine) and passive treatment (human or horse immune globulin) are used to prevent disease. If symptoms appear, essentially 100% fatality results. All other answer options are ineffective against rabies disease.

**96. The answer is a.** (*Brooks, pp 420–428. Levinson, pp 209–210, 255–256. Murray—2005, pp 553–559.*) Adenovirus type 8 is associated with epidemic keratoconjunctivitis, while adenovirus types 3 and 4 are often associated with "swimming pool conjunctivitis." There are also reports of nosocomial conjunctivitis with adenovirus. HSV can infect the conjunctiva and is among the most common causes of blindness in North America and Europe.

**97. The answer is a.** (*Brooks, pp 477–479. Levinson, pp 285–289. Murray—2005, pp 679, 684. Ryan, pp 547–549.*) The e antigen is related to the hepatitis B virus and is associated with viral replication (Dane particle). Possession of the e antigen suggests active disease and thus an increased risk of transmission of hepatitis to others. HBsAg and e antigen are components of hepatitis B only and are not shared by other hepatitis viruses.

**98. The answer is d.** (*Brooks, pp 514–519. Levinson, pp 294–295. Murray—2005, p 703. Ryan, p 586.*) Saint Louis encephalitis, yellow fever, and dengue are caused by flaviviruses. Western equine encephalitis is caused by an alphavirus. Laboratory diagnosis is usually made by demonstration of a four-fold rise in specific antibody titer in paired sera, although viruses may be isolated in specialist laboratories. Marburg virus and Ebola virus are filoviruses.

**99. The answer is e.** (*Brooks, pp 406, 560. Levinson, pp 233, 269. Murray—2005, pp 505, 509, 607. Ryan, pp 209–210.*) Ribavirin is effective to varying degrees against several RNA- and DNA-containing viruses in vitro. It has been approved for aerosol treatment of respiratory syncytial virus infections in infants. IV administration has proved effective in treating Lassa fever.

**100. The answer is c.** (*Brooks, pp 433–438. Murray—2005, pp 546–547. Ryan, pp 559–560.*) HSV causes primary and recurrent disease. The typical skin lesion is a vesicle that contains virus particles in serous fluid. Giant multinucleated cells are typically found at the base of the herpesvirus lesion. Encephalitis, which usually involves the temporal lobe, has a high mortality rate. Severe neurologic sequelae are seen in surviving patients. PCR amplification of viral DNA from CSF has replaced viral isolation.

**101. The answer is d.** (*Brooks, pp 446–449. Levinson, pp 250–251, 305. Murray—2005, pp 553–558. Ryan, pp 571–572.*) Contact with infected secretions such as saliva can result in infection with EBV, thus the term *kissing disease*. Laboratory diagnosis of EBV-induced infectious mononucleosis is usually determined by presence of atypical lymphocytes, heterophile antibodies, or specific antiviral antibodies such as VCA (viral capsid antibody).

**102. The answer is c.** (*Brooks, pp 558–560. Levinson, pp 267–268. Murray—2005, pp 606–607. Ryan, pp 504–506.*) RSV is the most important cause of pneumonia and bronchiolitis in infants. The infection is localized to the respiratory tract. The virus can be detected rapidly by immunofluorescence on smears of respiratory epithelium. In older children, the infection resembles the common cold. Aerosolized ribavirin is recommended for severely ill hospitalized infants. Wheezing symptoms observed in an RSV infection are most likely due to increased IgE antibodies. Adenoviruses and picornaviruses most often infect older children, not infants in this age range.

**103. The answer is b.** (*Brooks, pp 615–618. Levinson, pp 209, 313–321. Murray—2005, pp 665–667. Ryan, pp 609–610.*) Many believe that casual contact with patients who are HIV-positive increases the risk of acquiring the disease. This is not the case. It is also clear that homosexual females have a low rate of HIV acquisition. Because a substantial portion of the blood supply in Central African countries is HIV-infected, hospitalization is risky, particularly if transfusion is necessary.

**104. The answer is c.** (*Brooks, pp 566–568. Levinson, pp 269–270. Murray— 2005, pp 645–648. Ryan, pp 519–520.*) The highest risk of fetal infection with rubella occurs during the first trimester. In seronegative patients, the risk of infection exceeds 90%. However, before other measures (such as termination of pregnancy) are considered, a rubella immune status must be performed. A rubella titer of 1:10 is protective.

**105. The answer is a.** (*Brooks, pp 582–584. Levinson, pp 189–190, 308–312. Murray—2005, pp 691–694. Ryan, pp 627–628.*) Mad cow disease is related to both scrapie in sheep and bovine spongiform encephalopathy virus. The fear in Great Britain is the potential for acquiring CJD, which is a slowly progressive neurodegenerative disease. Theoretically, such acquisition could be through ingestion of beef from infected cows. A prion consists of protein material without nucleic acid. While related to a virus, a prion is a proteinaceous infectious particle that replicates within cells.

**106. The answer is d.** (*Brooks, p 470. Levinson, p 292. Murray—2005, p 689. Ryan, pp 552–553.*) HEV is a single-stranded RNA virus. It is transmitted enterically, and the disease is often referred to as *enteric hepatitis C*. There is no test for HEV routinely available. Diagnosis is clinical and is also one of exclusion. Rotavirus primarily affects children and not adults.

**107. The answer is e.** (*Brooks, pp 228, 707. Murray—2005, p 232. Ryan, p 501.*) *S. aureus* is the most common cause of postinfluenzal secondary bacterial pneumonia. It most often affects the elderly, although patients of any age may be afflicted. The pneumococcus as well as group A streptococci and *Haemophilus influenzae* may also cause pneumonia.

**108. The answer is a.** (*Brooks, pp 601–602. Murray—2005, pp 533–539.*) Conjunctivitis is inflammation of the eye tissue and is seen in many childhood infections. The most common cause, however, is infection with Adenoviruses. These also routinely cause URT and GI infections as well. Adenoviruses are easily spread between children, especially in community settings. Herpes simplex in the eye usually presents as a keratitis (corneal ulcer), with HSV1 occuring in adults and HSV2 in neonates. HSV most often occurs as a reactivation from a latent infection. S. aureus usually presents with a purulent discharge. *H. egypticus* may cause epidemic conjunctivitis but is usually seen in tropic climates. Trachoma (*C. trachomatis*) is most often seen in Africa, the Middle East, and nothern India. Transmitted by flies, fingers and fomites, repeated *C. trachomatis* infections may lead to blindness, although treatment with tetracycline or azithromycin can be curative.

**109. The answer is b.** (*Levinson, pp 215–216, p 322.*) In 1993, an outbreak of a fatal respiratory disease occurred in the southwestern United States. This disease is caused by a hantavirus endemic in deer mice. The mortality rate is 60%. Ribavirin has been used but is not effective. A vaccine is not available. Person-to-person transmission has been reported in South American outbreaks but is uncommon.

**110. The answer is a.** (*Brooks, pp 587–604. Levinson, pp 298–307. Murray—2005, pp 526–527. Ryan, pp 110–112.*) DNA tumor viruses encode viral oncoproteins that are important to viral replication but also affect cellular growth control pathways. Most RNA tumor viruses belong to the retrovirus family, carrying a reverse transcriptase enzyme (RNA-dependent DNA polymerase) that is responsible for contructing a DNA copy of the viral RNA genome. Direct-transforming RNA oncoviruses carry an oncogene of cellular origin, whereas weakly oncogenic RNA viruses have no oncogene and produce leukemias after long incubation periods by indirect mechanisms.

| ASSOCIATION OF VIRUSES WITH HUMAN CANCERS.* | | |
| Virus Family | Virus | Human Cancer |
| --- | --- | --- |
| Papovaviridae | Human papillo-<br>maviruses | Genital tumors<br>Squamous cell carcinoma<br>Oropharyngeal carcinoma |
| Herpesviridae | EB virus | Nasopharyngeal carcinoma<br>African Burkitt's lymphoma<br>B-cell lymphoma |
| Hepadnaviridae | Hepatitis B virus | Hepatocellular carcinoma |
| Retroviridae | HTL virus | Adult T cell leukemia |
| Flaviviridae | Hepatitis C virus | Hepatocellular carcinoma |

*Candidate human tumor viruses include human herpesvirus 8, additional types of papillomaviruses, and human and simian polyomaviruses.

*Reprinted, with permission, from Brooks GF et al.* Jawetz's Medical Microbiology, 22e. *New York: McGraw-Hill, 2001.*

**111. The answer is d.** (*Brooks, pp 599–601. Levinson, pp 298–307. Murray— 2005, pp 523–527.*) Only two human viruses have been confirmed as human tumor viruses. They include human T cell lymphotrophic/leukemia virus (HTLV) and papillomavirus. Others, such as EBV, HSV, and hepatitis B and C, have been implicated as tumor viruses. The virus that causes chickenpox and shingles (VZV) is not known to be oncogenic.

**112. The answer is a.** (*Brooks, pp 420–428. Levinson, pp 255–256, 257–258. Murray—2005, pp 533–539. Ryan, pp 522–523.*) Adenoviruses are widespread and cause a variety of respiratory and gastrointestinal clinical problems. Many of the "viral sore throats" among young people living in close quarters are due to adenovirus. Parvovirus B19, not adenovirus, causes acute hemolytic anemia.

**113. The answer is a.** (*Brooks, pp 442–446. Levinson, pp 249–250. Murray— 2005, pp 558–561. Ryan, pp 567–568.*) Although infection with CMV is common, it only rarely causes clinically apparent disease. Lesions characteristic of infection with CMV are found in up to 10% of stillborn babies; however, CMV, which can be transmitted transplacentally, usually is not the cause of death. Children and adults with immunosuppressive problems are susceptible to active disease. In severely immunodeficient patients such as those with AIDS, CMV ocular disease may occur. The patient suffers blurring of vision or vision loss, and ophthalmic examination reveals large yellowish-white areas with flame-shaped hemorrhages. Ganciclovir is now licensed for treatment of CMV retinitis in AIDS patients. CMV was one of the first viruses shown to be capable of causing in utero infection.

**114. The answer is d.** *(Brooks, pp 505–508. Levinson, pp 281, 509. Murray—2005, pp 627–633. Ryan, pp 578–580.)* Rotaviruses were initially identified by direct electron microscopy (EM) of duodenal mucosa of infants with gastroenteritis. Subsequent studies in several countries have shown them to be the cause of 30–40% of cases of acute diarrhea in infants. They are nonlipid-containing RNA viruses with a double-shelled capsid. Although the virus has been serially propagated in human fetal intestinal organ cultures, cytopathic changes are minimal or absent; multiplication is detected by immunofluorescence. Numerous methods for rotavirus antigen detection, including radioimmunoassay, counterimmunoelectrophoresis, and ELISA, have been developed and found to be about as effective as EM.

**115. The answer is d.** *(Brooks, pp 562–564. Levinson, p 309. Murray—2005, pp 598–603. Ryan, pp 517–518.)* SSPE is a late and rare manifestation of measles. It is a progressive encephalitis involving both white and gray matter. Demyelination is seen only at an advanced stage of the disease in a few cases. In 1985, viral RNA was demonstrated in brain cells from a patient with SSPE by the use of in situ hybridization.

**116. The answer is b.** *(Brooks, pp 505–508. Levinson, pp 281, 509. Murray—2005, pp 627–633. Ryan, pp 578–580.)* Rotavirus is a viral entity that is similar to Nebraska calf diarrhea virus and is thought to be a major cause of acute diarrhea in newborn infants. Three-quarters of all adults have antibodies against rotavirus; passive transfer of these antibodies to the baby, especially through the colostrum, seems to be protective. Although vaccination would be expected to be of little use to the neonate, it might effectively immunize pregnant mothers.

**117. The answer is a.** *(Brooks, pp 561–566. Levinson, pp 264–268. Murray—2005, pp 598–606. Ryan, pp 506–507.)* Both mumps and measles are well-recognized paramyxovirus infections. This group also includes parainfluenza virus, which causes laryngotracheobronchitis (croup) in children, and respiratory syncytial virus, which can cause bronchiolitis in infants. Paramyxoviruses have glycoprotein spikes that extend their lipid membrane and are responsible for hemagglutination activities.

**118. The answer is a.** (*Brooks, pp 447–448. Murray—2005, p 562.*) Aggressive monoclonal B-cell lymphomas can develop in patients with reduced T-cell function. The immortalization of B-cells in the absence of functional T-cell immunity can give rise to lymphoproliferative disease such as Hodgkin's lymphoma, Burkitt's lymphoma and nasopharyngeal carcinoma.

**119. The answer is c.** (*Brooks, p 713. Levinson, pp 272–274. Murray—2005, pp 505, 681. Ryan, p 545.*) The replication of a retroviral genome is dependent on the reverse transcriptase enzyme, which performs a variety of functions. It builds a complementary strand of DNA from the viral RNA template; it builds a second DNA strand complementary to the previous DNA; it degrades the original RNA, leaving a DNA–DNA duplex; and, finally, it is responsible for integrating the new viral DNA hybrid into the host genome.

**120. The answer is c.** (*Brooks, pp 514–519. Levinson, pp 294–296. Murray—2005, p 703. Ryan, p 591.*) Saint Louis encephalitis virus has structural and biologic characteristics in common with other Flaviviruses. It is the most important arboviral disease in North America. Saint Louis encephalitis virus was first isolated from mosquitoes in California. Patients who contract the disease usually present with one of three clinical manifestations: febrile headache, aseptic meningitis, or clinical encephalitis.

**121. The answer is c.** (*Brooks, pp 442–446. Levinson, pp 249–250. Murray—2005, pp 558–561. Ryan, p 568.*) (See figure.) Presently, cytomegalovirus (CMV) is the most common cause of congenital and perinatal viral infections. Culture of the virus is a sensitive diagnostic technique; in the case of a neonate with classic symptoms, serum samples from the mother and neonate are obtained at birth. The IgM antibody titer in the infant's serum should be higher than the mother's titer, but they may be similar. For this reason, another sample from the infant at one month of age is tested simultaneously with the initial sample. The results should indicate a rise in IgM titer. Measurement of total IgM in the infant's sera at birth is nonspecific and may show false-negative and false-positive reactions.

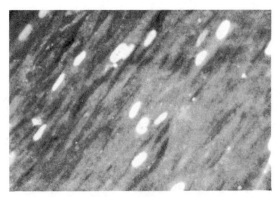

Cytomegalovirus-infected human embryonic fibroblasts stained with fluorescein-labeled monoclonal antibody to early nuclear antigen (×1000).

**122. The answer is e.** *(Brooks, pp 406–408. Levinson, pp 221–222, 234. Murray—2005, pp 144–146. Ryan, pp 104, 212.)* IFN is a protein that alters cell metabolism to inhibit viral replication. It induces the formation of a second protein that interferes with the translation of viral messenger RNA. Production of IFN has been demonstrated when cells in tissue culture are challenged with viruses, rickettsiae, endotoxin, or synthetic double-stranded polynucleotides. IFN confers species-specific, not virus-specific, protection for cells.

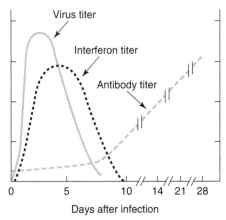

Illustration of kinetics of interferon and antibody synthesis after respiratory viral infection. The temporal relationships suggest that interferons are involved in the recovery process. *(Reproduced, with permission, from Brooks GF et al. Jawetz's Medical Microbiology, 22e. New York: McGraw-Hill, 2001.)*

**123. The answer is e.** *(Brooks, pp 466–467. Murray—2005, pp 677–678.)* Since this was diagnosed and confirmed as a Hepatitis A infection, there is little likelyhood of long term sequelae. One dose of standard gamma globulin, which contains antibodies from a series of normal population individuals, will provide passive protection to the family members for several weeks due to the presence of antibodies against HAV. Vaccination with the killed HAV vaccine might be considered, but for immediate protection, the preformed anti–HAV antibodies will provide immediate and excellent protection. HAV transmits readily, so the no-treatment option could not guarantee no transmission might occur within the family. IFN treatment is approved only for HBV and HCV infections.

**124. The answer is e.** *(Brooks, pp 446–449. Levinson, pp 250–251, 305. Murray—2005, pp 553–558. Ryan, p 472.)* With an acute case of primary infection by EBV, such as infectious mononucleosis, IgM antibodies to VCA should be present. Antibodies to EBNA should be absent, as they usually appear 2–3 months after onset of illness. Culture is not clinically useful because it (1) requires freshly fractionated cord blood lymphocytes, (2) takes 3–4 weeks for completion, and (3) is reactive in the majority of seropositive patients.

**125. The answer is a.** *(Brooks, pp 420–428. Levinson, pp 244–252, 255–256. Murray—2005, pp 533–539. Ryan, p 508.)* While the herpesviruses (HSV, CMV, VZV) are all well known for latency, adenovirus can also form a latent infection in the lymphoid tissue. In 50–80% of surgically removed tonsils or adenoids, adenovirus can be cultured. The virus has also been cultured from mesenteric lymph nodes, and, in rare cases, viral DNA has been detected in peripheral lymphocytes. Recurrent illness usually does not arise from these latent infections; however, activation can occur in the immunosuppressed.

**126. The answer is b.** *(Brooks, pp 542–547. Levinson, pp 259–264. Murray— 2005, pp 611–615. Ryan, p 501.)* The symptoms described are consistent with influenza virus infection. The titers of antibody on November 6 and 30 show low levels of antibody against swine influenza, but indicate at least a measurable amount. The 160 titer on December 20 reflects a definitive diagnostic rise in antibody against swine influenza (>1:4 rise between acute and convalescent sera).

The previous titers (10 or 1:10) most likely represent cross-reacting antibodies from a non-swine influenza virus hemagglutinin or neuraminidase enzymes, which could account for cross-reacting antibodies.

**127. The answer is c.** *(Brooks, pp 446–449. Levinson, pp 250–251, 305. Murray—2005, pp 553–558. Ryan, p 572.)* EBV replication initially occurs in epithelial cells of the pharynx and salivary glands. Infected B cells spread the infection systematically. Most virus-infected cells are eliminated in healthy hosts, but small numbers may persist for a lifetime. Atypical lymphocytes are the hematologic hallmark of infectious mononucleosis with 90% or more of the circulating lymphocytes being atypical in some cases. These abnormal lymphocytes are not pathognomonic for infectious mononucleosis. They are also seen in other diseases, including CMV infection, viral hepatitis, toxoplasmosis, rubella, mumps, and roseola.

**128. The answer is a.** *(Brooks, pp 526–527. Levinson, pp 211, 297. Murray—2005, p 644. Ryan, p 592.)* Dengue (breakbone fever) is caused by a group B togavirus that is transmitted by mosquitoes. The clinical syndrome usually consists of a mild systemic disease characterized by severe joint and muscle pain, headache, fever, lymphadenopathy, and a maculopapular rash. Hemorrhagic dengue, a more severe syndrome, may be prominent during some epidemics; shock and, occasionally, death result.

**129. The answer is e.** *(Brooks, pp 469–470. Levinson, pp 289–291. Murray—2005, pp 685–687. Ryan, pp 551–552.)* HCV is a positive-stranded RNA virus, classified as a flavivirus. About half of HCV patients develop chronic hepatitis. A large number of infections appear among IV drug abusers. About 90% of the cases of transfusion-associated hepatitis are thought to be caused by HCV.

**130–133. The answers are 130-c, 131-e, 132-b, 133-a.** *(Brooks, pp 470–484. Levinson, pp 283–292. Murray—2005, pp 678–680. Ryan, pp 548–549.)* Advances in the serodiagnosis of viral hepatitis have been dramatic, and the findings of specific viral antigens have led to further elucidation of the course of infections. The "Australia antigen," discovered in 1960, was first renamed hepatitis-associated antigen (HAA) and then, finally, hepatitis B surface antigen (HBsAg). It appears in the blood early after infection, before onset of acute illness, and persists through early convalescence.

HBsAg usually disappears within 4–6 months after the start of clinical illness, except in the case of chronic carriers.

HBeAg appears during the early acute phase and disappears before HBsAg is gone, although it may persist in the chronic carrier. Persons who are HBeAg-positive have higher titers of HBV and therefore are at a higher risk of transmitting the disease. HBeAg has a high correlation with DNA polymerase activity.

The HBcAg is found within the nuclei of infected hepatocytes and not generally in the peripheral circulation except as an integral component of the Dane particle. The antibody to this antigen, anti–HBc, is present at the beginning of clinical illness. As long as there is ongoing HBV replication, there will be high titers of anti–HBc. During the early convalescent phase of an HBV infection, anti–HBc may be the only detectable serologic marker (window phase) if HBsAg is negative and anti–HBsAg has not appeared.

**134–138. The answers are 134-a, 135-b, 136-c, 137-c, 138-e.** (*Brooks, pp 442–446, 540, 575–581. Levinson, pp 249–250, 266–267, 259, 271–272, 275–280. Murray—2005, pp 559–561, 611–615, 621–622. Ryan, pp 510, 503–505, 513–514, 567–568, 598.*) CMV causes cytomegalic inclusion disease (CID), especially congenital abnormalities, in neonates. Malformations include microencephaly. Seizures, deafness, jaundice, and purpura can also occur. CID is also one of the leading causes of mental retardation in the United States. Orchitis, a complication of mumps virus infection in postpubertal males, can cause sterility if bilateral. Antigenic drift and antigenic shift account for antigenic changes in the two surface glycoproteins (HA-hemeagglutin and NA-neuraminadase) of influenza viruses. Antigenic drift is a gradual change in antigenicity due to point mutations that affect major antigenic sites on the glycoprotein. Antigenic shift is an abrupt change due to genetic reassortment with an unrelated strain of virus. Changes in HA and NA occur independently. Internal proteins of the virus (NP, for example) do not undergo antigenic changes. The rabies virus is transmitted by the bite of a rabid animal. It almost always causes a fatal encephalitis if untreated. Postexposure treatment includes use of a killed vaccine and human rabies globulin (HIG). While HIV can cross the placenta, it results in infection with no malformations as described. Rubeola (measles) does not cross the placenta, ehile Rubells (German measles) can. Rubella is also responsible for a wide range of in utero malformations. Rubeola (measles) is also a paramyxovirus, but does not cause complications with the testes or ovaries.

**139–143. The answers are 139-c, 140-b, 141-d, 142-a, 143-d.** *(Brooks, pp 466–469, 542–547, 438, 466–467. Levinson, pp 283–284, 259–264, 261–262, 229, 231, 239. Murray—2005, pp 678–685, 611–615, 507–508, 675–678. Ryan, pp 502–503, 518, 544, 549, 561–562.)* The original vaccine for hepatitis B was prepared by purifying hepatitis B surface antigen (HBsAg) from healthy HBsAg-positive carriers and treating it with viral-inactivating agents. The second-generation vaccine for hepatitis B is produced by recombinant DNA in yeast cells containing a plasmid into which the gene for HBsAg has been incorporated.

Influenza usually occurs in successive waves of infection with peak incidences during the winter months. If only minor antigenic drift is expected for the next influenza season, then the most recent strains of A and B viruses representative of the main antigens are included in the vaccine. Influenza vaccine consists of killed viruses.

Live attenuated measles virus vaccine effectively prevents measles. Protection is provided if given before or within 2 days of exposure. Vaccination confers immunity for at least 15 years.

Acyclovir is an analogue of guanosine or deoxyguanosine that strongly inhibits HSV but has little effect on other DNA viruses. When employed for the treatment of primary genital infection by HSV, both oral and IV formulations have reduced viral shedding and shortened the duration of symptoms.

The vaccine for HAV is prepared from virus grown in culture and inactivated with formalin. Passive immunization with immune serum globulin confers passive protection in 90% of those exposed when given within 1–2 weeks after exposure.

**144–148. The answers are 144-e, 145-a, 146-c, 147-d, 148-c.** *(Brooks, pp 438–440, 420–428, 599–601, 562–566, 442–446. Levinson, pp 248–249, 249–250, 255–256, 256–257, 281. Murray—2005, pp 550–553, 533–539, 523–524, 597, 559–561. Ryan, pp 509–510, 564–565, 568, 579, 619.)* Varicella- zoster virus is a herpesvirus. Chickenpox is a highly contagious disease of childhood that occurs in the late winter and early spring. It is characterized by a generalized vesicular eruption with relatively insignificant systemic manifestations.

Adenovirus has been associated with adult respiratory disease among newly enlisted military troops. Crowded conditions and strenuous exercise may account for the severe infections seen in this otherwise healthy group.

Papillomavirus is one of two members of the family Papovaviridae, which includes viruses that produce human warts. These viruses are host-specific and produce benign epithelial tumors that vary in location and clinical appearance. The warts usually occur in children and young adults and are limited to the skin and mucous membranes.

Rubeola (measles) virus produces a maculopapular rash. No vesicles or pustule forms are developed and no successive crops of lesions are formed.

Infectious mononucleosis caused by CMV is clinically difficult to distinguish from that caused by EBV. Lymphocytosis is usually present, with an abundance of atypical lymphocytes. CMV-induced mononucleosis should be considered in any case of mononucleosis that is heterophil-negative and in patients with fever of unknown origin.

**149–153. The answers are 149-b, 150-b, 151-c, 152-a, 153-a.** *(Brooks, pp 446–449, 729. Levinson, pp 250–251, 305, 438, 440, 249–250. Murray—2005, pp 553–558, 188. Ryan, pp 515–518, 569–572, 724.)* EBV is a herpesvirus that causes a number of syndromes; the most common is infectious mononucleosis. It is a ubiquitous enveloped DNA virus. Only one serotype of EBV has been recognized, although molecular methods have reorganized a number of genotypes of EBV.

Complement fixation antibody measurements against viruses may be a useful diagnostic tool if two serum samples are collected from the patient. The acute serum is collected as early in the illness as possible, and the convalescent serum is collected 7–10 days later. Both are included in the same test run against measles CF antigen. A positive diagnostic test occurs in the antibody titer when the convalescent serum is fourfold or greater than the acute sample. The sera are diluted in a twofold manner (1:2, 1:4, 1:8, and so on) for quantitation. The measures given above (40 and 80) are considered essentially the same level of antibodies in both samples. This patient must have had measles in the past and has the same amount of antibody in both serum samples.

Infectious mononucleosis is an acute disease most commonly seen in younger people. It is characterized by a proliferation of lymphocytes, lymph node enlargement, pharyngitis, fatigue, and fever. Infection in young children is usually either asymptomatic or characteristic of an acute upper respiratory infection. Diagnosis is usually made by a positive heterophil test. Heterophil antibodies are those that occur in one species (human) and react with antigens of a different species. The heterophil test may be insensitive (30–60%) in children. Definitive diagnosis is made by detection of antibodies to EBV components. EBV causes a variety of other syndromes including Burkitt's lymphoma, the most common childhood cancer in Africa, and nasopharyngeal carcinoma, commonly seen in China. Similar mononucleosis-like diseases are caused by CMV and *Toxoplasma gondii*, a parasite. CMV causes fewer than 10% of infectious mononucleosis-like diseases. CMV "mono" is primarily characterized by fatigue. Congenital infection with CMV almost always causes serious sequelae, such as retardation and hearing loss. *T. gondii* also causes a variety of clinical problems, among them encephalitis in AIDS patients and food poisoning from the ingestion of raw meat. Although CMV and *T. gondii* are relatively rare causes of infectious mononucleosis, they must be ruled out, particularly when EBV tests are nonreactive.

**154–158. The answers are 154-b, 155-a, 156-b, 157-d, 158-d.** *(Brooks, pp 731–734, 391. Murray—2005, pp 513–521. Ryan, p 231.)* The diagnosis of a viral infection is made easier by the creation of a greater number of diagnostic virology laboratories during the past few decades. In order for viral diagnosis to be successful, the most appropriate specimen must be collected for the disease in question.

HPV is often detected microscopically in cervical biopsies. Alternatively, there are methods to detect HPV DNA in such tissues as well as to serotype the virus. Evidence suggests that some HPV serotypes are more likely than others to cause cervical cancer.

Many viruses have a viremic phase, but only a few, such as CMV, persist after the patient becomes symptomatic. CMV can be isolated from lymphocytes and polymorphonuclear leukocytes. This usually requires special separation procedures, particularly in those compromised patients who may be neutropenic.

Enteroviruses such as echoviruses and coxsackieviruses are the predominant cause of aseptic viral meningitis. While enterovirus infections are often diagnosed by specific antibody response, it is possible to isolate the virus from CSF. HSV can also be isolated from CSF in cases of herpes encephalitis or meningitis.

VZV and HSV are most often recovered from skin lesions, although varicella IgM antibody detection may be the most rapid way to diagnose acute VZV infection. Detection and identification of these viruses is essential because of the availability of antiviral agents such as acyclovir. Other viruses, such as enteroviruses and paramyxoviruses, cause skin lesions.

Many viruses can be isolated from feces. Of the viral groups in these questions, adenovirus 40/41 is the most common stool isolate. Norwalk agent and other caliciviruses may also be isolated or detected from stools, but usually only in specialized laboratories.

**159–163. The answers are 159-c, 160-a, 161-e, 162-d, 163-b.** *(Brooks, pp 774–775. Murray—2005, pp 84–85. Ryan, p 578.)* A number of viruses that cause gastroenteritis are now being recognized. The following table summarizes the characteristics of rotavirus, Norwalk virus, adenovirus, calicivirus, and astrovirus. (see table, p. XXX.)

**164. The answer is e.** *(Brooks, pp 566–568. Murray—2005, pp 644–648.)* Rubella (German measles, 3 day measles) is an acute febrile illness characterized by a rash and lymphadenopathy that affects children and young adults. It is the mildest of the viral examthems. Problems arise from in utero infections, especially within the first trimester of pregnancy, when serious and permanent damage, including fatalities, may occur in the fetus. The incubation period is average for viral infections, approximately 1 week. The infections are controlled within the population by using an excellent live, attenuated vaccine. Rubella is an excellent antigen, giving rise to antibodies that provide essentially lifelong protection against the wild type virus. These preexisting antibodies have been shown to be the main mechanism of protection. Koplik's spots are characteristic of rubeola (hard measles) infection. Rubella is classified as part of the Togavirus group, while rubeola is a paramyxovirus.

**165–168. The answers are 165-c, 166-b, 167-e, 168-d.** *(Brooks, pp 470–484. Levinson, pp 283–292. Murray—2005, pp 676–685. Ryan, p 542.)* Hepatitis A virus (HAV) possesses a single-stranded linear RNA genome, while hepatitis B virus (HBV) contains a double-stranded DNA genome. Detection of anti–HAV IgM in a single serum specimen obtained in the acute or convalescent stage is the quickest and most reliable method to diagnose hepatitis A infection. This antibody is usually present at onset of symptoms and may persist 3–6 months. Demonstration of hepatitis B surface antigen (HBsAg) in serum is the most common method of diagnosing HBV infection. Other serologic markers helpful in characterizing infection with HBV include hepatitis B surface antibody (anti–HBs), anti–hepatitis B core (anti–HBc), anti-hepatitis B e antigen (anti–HBe), and hepatitis B e

| | Norwalk and Norwalk-like Viruses | Rotavirus | Others | | |
|---|---|---|---|---|---|
| | | | Adenovirus | Calicivirus | Astrovirus |
| Size (nm) diameter | 27–35 | 70 | 70–90 | 35–39 | 27–35 |
| Nucleic acid | RNA (single-stranded) | RNA (double-stranded) | DNA | RNA | RNA |
| Minimum number of serotypes | 3 | 4 (3 groups, A, B, C) | 2 | 3–5 | 5 |
| Seasonality (temperate climate) | Winter | Winter | All seasons | — | — |
| Epidemicity | Epidemic | Sporadic, epidemic | Sporadic | Epidemic | Sporadic |
| Age with clinical disease | ≥6 yr | 6–24 mo most common | ≤2 yr | ≤2 yr | ≤7 yr |
| Transmission | Fecal-oral, water, food | Fecal-oral, water, food | Fecal-oral | Fecal-oral | Fecal-oral |

*Adapted, with permission, from Howard BJ, Keiser JF, Smith TF, Weissfeld AS, Tilton RC: Clinical and Pathogenic Microbiology, 2/e, St. Louis, Mosby, 1993.*

antigen (HBeAg). Several epidemiologic studies have demonstrated that immune serum globulin (ISG) can prevent clinical hepatitis A even when given up to 10 days after exposure. Similar studies have shown that ISG was able to decrease the incidence of hepatitis B infection in exposed persons. Purified, noninfectious HBsAg derived from healthy HBsAg carriers has been used as a vaccine for active immunization for HBV infection. Hepatitis C is a single-stranded RNA virus belonging to the family Flaviviridae. The viral reservoir is human. Recent retrospective "lookbacks" suggest that many people were infected with HCV before testing of the blood supply was initiated in the early 1990s. HCV is treatable with combinations of drugs. The genotype of the virus plays an important role in the determination of length of therapy. Hepatitis D virus is an incomplete or defective virus that requires HBsAg as a cofactor. Both coinfection and secondary delta infection exist, with secondary infection being the most serious. Hepatitis E virus is an RNA virus. Transmission is by the fecal-oral route, although maternal-fetal transmission has recently been described. Prognosis is usually favorable with rare cases of fulminant HEV reported.

**169. The answer is b.** (*Brooks, pp 491–499. Levinson, pp 275–279. Murray—2005, pp 583–586. Ryan, pp 532–535.*) Enteroviruses (polio-, Coxsackie-, and echoviruses) are ingested in contaminated water and/or food. Their main replication occurs in the intestinal tract, and virus progeny may get into the blood. From blood, distant target organs (the CNS, for example) may become involved. Most enterovirus CNS infections are self-limited, but some may progress to a life-threatening stage. Mumps virus and coronaviruses are inhaled initially. Influenza does not replicate in lymphocytes and does not involve the CNS. HIV has not been shown to be transmitted by any type of insect vector.

**170–172. The answers are 170-e, 171-b, 172-b.** (*Brooks, pp 597–601, 433. Levinson, pp 296, 209, 306, 244–255. Murray—2005, pp 523–532, 541. Ryan pp 559–561.*) West Nile virus (WNV) is an arbovirus. Although prevalent in Europe, Africa, and the Middle East, it was not seen in the United States until the summer of 1999. It is transmitted by mosquitoes and birds, especially crows; these animals are a reservoir. WNV causes a rather mild encephalitis in humans, the exception being older patients or those who may be immunocompromised.

Although most infections by HPV are benign, some undergo malignant transformation into in situ and invasive squamous cell carcinoma. Both HPV and polyomavirus have icosahedral capsids and DNA genomes. JC virus, a polyomavirus, was first isolated from the diseased brain of a patient with Hodgkin's lymphoma who was dying of progressive multifocal PML. This demyelinating disease occurs usually in immunosuppressed persons and is the result of oligodendrocyte infection by JC virus. JC virus has also been isolated from the urine of patients suffering from demyelinating disease. Cryotherapy and laser treatment are the most popular therapies for warts, although surgery may be indicated in some cases. At the present time, there is no effective antiviral therapy for treatment of infection with polyomavirus or HPV.

Primary HSV-1 infections are usually asymptomatic. Symptomatic disease occurs most frequently in small children (1–5 years old). Buccal and gingival mucosa are most often involved, and lesions, if untreated, may last 2–3 weeks. Acyclovir treatment is effective therapy and should be started immediately. The classic location of latent HSV-1 infection is the trigeminal ganglia. Reactivation results in sporadic vesicular lesions and may also be treated with acyclovir. B cell activation would be unusual, and there appears to be no greater risk for cancer development than that seen in the general population.

**173. The answer is e.** (*Brooks, pp 453–465. Levinson, pp 252–253. Murray—2005, pp 565–571.*) The disease is caused by Molluscum contagiosum, a Poxvirus. It is characterized by small white papules with a central depression and usually found in the genital region. HPV cause genital warts but differ in the type of lesions described in the clinical situation. Adenoviruses cause a variety of infections, including respiratory, ocular, and GI diseases. Parvoviruses and Arenaviruses do not produce lesions described in the question.

**174–177. The answers are 174-c, 175-e, 176-d, 177-a.** (*Brooks, pp 453–465, 550–566. Levinson, pp 261–262, 267–268, 255–256. Murray—2005, pp 565–571, 597–608. Ryan, pp 499–511.*) The paramyxoviruses include several important human pathogens (mumps virus, measles virus, respiratory syncytial virus, and parainfluenza virus). Both paramyxoviruses and orthomyxoviruses possess an RNA-dependent RNA polymerase that is a structural component of the virion and produces the initial RNA. RSVs are not related to the paramyxoviruses. They are 150-nm single-stranded RNA viruses. There are two antigen groups, A and B, which play no role in diagnosis and treatment. While the overall mortality rate is 0.5%, for at-risk groups mortality may be 25–35% if untreated. Some parainfluenza virus infections (type 3) may be indistinguishable from RSV, but most parainfluenza infections produce a laryngotracheobronchitis known as croup. Mumps, measles, variola (smallpox), and coronaviruses all exhibit definite viremic stages in their infections. RSV, on the other hand, is the most important cause of lower respiratory tract illness in infants. RSV is inhaled and viral replication occurs initially in the epithelial cells of the nasopharynx. From there, it may spread to the lower respiratory tract, causing bronchoiolitis or pneumonia. The virus remains localized and is isolated from bronchial wash materials or identified in exfoliated epithelial cells, indicating the relative lack of a viremic stage. Current treatment, in fact, consists of ribovirin being delivered in an aerosol format.

# Bacteriology

## Questions

**DIRECTIONS:**   Each question below contains four or more suggested responses. Select the **one best** response to each question.

**178.** A patient with a burning epigastric pain was admitted to the hospital, and a gastric biopsy was performed. The tissue was cultured on chocolate agar incubated in a microaerophilic environment at 37°C for 5–7 days. At 5 days of incubation, colonies appeared on the plate and curved, gram-negative rods, oxidase-positive, were observed. Which of the following is the most likely identity of this organism?

a.  *Campylobacter fetus*
b.  *Campylobacter jejuni*
c.  *Haemophilus influenzae*
d.  *Helicobacter pylori*
e.  *Vibrio parahaemolyticus*

**179.** A 2-year-old boy who missed several scheduled immunizations presents to the emergency room with a high fever, irritability, and a stiff neck. Fluid from a spinal tap reveals 20,000 white blood cells WBCs per mL with 85% polymorphonuclear cells. Gram stain evaluation of the fluid reveals small pleomorphic gram-negative rods that grow on chocolate agar. If an inhibitor is designed to block its major virulence, which of the following would be the most likely target?

a.  Capsule formation
b.  Endotoxin assembly
c.  Exotoxin liberator
d.  Flagella synthesis
e.  IgA protease synthesis

**180.** An experimental compound is discovered that prevents the activation of adenylate cyclase and the resulting increase in cyclic AMP. The toxic effects of which of the following bacteria would most likely be prevented with the use of this experimental compound?

a. *Brucella abortus*
b. *Corynebacterium diphtheriae*
c. *Listeria monocytogenes*
d. *Pseudomonas aeruginosa*
e. *Vibrio cholerae*

**181.** A single, 30-year-old woman presents to her physician with vaginitis. She complains of a slightly increased, malodorous discharge that is gray-white in color, thin, and homogenous. Clue cells are discovered when the discharge is examined microscopically. Which of the following organisms is the most likely cause of her infection?

a. *Candida albicans*
b. *Trichomonas vaginalis*
c. *Escherichia coli*
d. *Gardnerella vaginalis*
e. *Staphylococcus aureus*

**182.** A 12-year-old girl was playing soccer when she began to limp. She has pain in her right leg and upper right thigh. Her temperature is 102°F. X-ray of the femur reveals that the periosteum is eroded. Which of the following is the most likely etiologic agent?

a. *L. monocytogenes*
b. *Salmonella enteritidis*
c. *Staphylococcus saprophyticus*
d. *S. aureus*
e. *Streptococcus pneumoniae*

**183.** A scraping from a painful, inflamed wound is found to contain numerous gram-negative bacteria. Upon questioning, the feverish patient states that he was bitten by a cat while trying to rescue it from a storm drain earlier in the day. Given these observations, which of the following organisms is the most likely cause of infection?

a. *Aeromonas* species
b. *C. jejuni*
c. *Pasteurella multocida*
d. *Pseudomonas aeruginosa*
e. *Yersinia enterocolitica*

## Item 184–186

A 21-year-old college student complains of malaise, low-grade fever, and a harsh cough, but not of muscle aches and pains. An x-ray reveals a diffuse interstitial pneumonia in the left lobes of the lung. The WBC count is normal. The student has been ill for a week.

**184.** Which of the following is the most likely diagnosis?

a. Influenza
b. Legionellosis
c. Mycoplasma pneumonia
d. Pneumococcal pneumonia
e. Staphylococcal pneumonia

**185.** Which of the following laboratory tests would most rapidly assist the physician in making the diagnosis?

a. Cold agglutinins
b. Complement fixation (CF) test
c. Culture of sputum
d. Gram stain of sputum
e. Viral culture

**186.** The following laboratory data were available within 2 days: cold agglutinins—negative; complement fixation (*Mycoplasma pneumoniae*)—1:64; viral culture—pending, but negative to date; bacterial culture of sputum on blood agar and MacConkey's agar—normal oral flora. In order to confirm the diagnosis, which of the following procedures should be ordered to achieve a specific and sensitive diagnosis?

a.  A DNA probe to the 16S ribosomal RNA of an organism lacking a cell wall
b.  Another viral culture in 1 week
c.  A repeat CF test in 5 days
d.  A repeat cold agglutinin test
e.  Culture of the sputum on charcoal yeast extract

**187.** A 40-year-old male had been in good health until he began experiencing a chronic cough. Over the following 6 weeks the cough gradually worsened and became productive. He also noted weight loss, fever, night sweats, and coughing blood. A sputum sample was positive for acid-fast bacilli. Which of the following pathogenic mechanisms can be primarily attributed to the etiologic agent involved in this disease?

a.  Cell-mediated hypersensitivity
b.  Clogging of alveoli by large numbers of acid-fast mycobacteria
c.  Humoral immunity
d.  Specific cell adhesion sites
e.  Toxin production by the mycobacteria

**188.** The class of antibiotics known as the quinolones is bactericidal. Which of the following is the best characterization of their mode of action on growing bacteria?

a.  Inactivation of penicillin-binding protein II
b.  Inhibition of β-lactamase
c.  Inhibition of DNA gyrase
d.  Inhibition of reverse transcriptase
e.  Prevention of the cross-linking of glycine

**189.** Vancomycin-indeterminate *S. aureus* (VISA) has recently been reported in the United States. Which of the following statements concerning VISA is correct?

a. Patients with VISA isolates need not be isolated
b. Minimum inhibitory concentration (MIC) for vancomycin is at least 1.0 mcg/mL
c. VISAs have emerged because of the extended use of vancomycin for methicillin-resistant *S. aureus* (MRSAs)
d. VISA isolates are infrequent, so surveillance at the present time is not warranted
e. VISA isolates are usually methicillin susceptible

**190.** A 3-year-old girl, who has missed several scheduled immunizations, presents to the emergency room with a fever trouble breathing. A sputum sample is brought to the laboratory for analysis. Gram stain reveals the following: rare epithelial cells, 8–10 polymorphonuclear leukocytes per high-power field, and pleomorphic gram-negative rods. As a laboratory consultant, which of the following interpretations is correct?

a. The appearance of the sputum is suggestive of *H. influenzae*
b. The patient has pneumococcal pneumonia
c. The patient has Vincent's disease
d. The sputum specimen is too contaminated by saliva to be useful
e. There is no evidence of an inflammatory response

**191.** A 25-year-old medical student presented with a ruptured appendix. A peritoneal infection developed, despite prompt removal of the organ and extensive flushing of the peritoneal cavity. An isolate from a pus culture was a gram-negative rod identified as *Bacteroides fragilis*. Anaerobic infection with *B. fragilis* is best characterized by which of the following?

a. A black exudate in the wound
b. A foul-smelling discharge
c. A heme-pigmented colony formation
d. An exquisite susceptibility to penicillin
e. Severe neurologic symptoms

**192.** Several days after an unprotected sexual encounter, a healthy 21-year-old male develops pain and pus on urination. A Gram stain reveals gram-negative diplococci. Which of the following structures is responsible for adherence of the offending microbe to the urethral mucosa?

a. Capsule
b. Fimbriae
c. Flagella
d. The F pili
e. The peptidoglycan
f. The lipopolysaccharide (LPS)

**193.** A 4-week-old newborn develops meningitis. Short, gram-positive rods are isolated. History reveals that the mother had eaten unpasteurized cheese from Mexico during the pregnancy, and she recalled having a flulike illness. Which of the following is the most likely etiologic microorganism?

a. *C. diphtheriae*
b. *E. coli*
c. Group B streptococci
d. *L. monocytogenes*
e. *S. pneumoniae*

### Questions 194–197

**194.** A 30-year-old male patient is seen by the emergency service and reports a 2-week history of a penile ulcer. He notes that this ulcer did not hurt. Which of the following conclusions/actions is most valid?

a. Draw blood for a herpes antibody test
b. Even if treated, the lesion will remain for months
c. Failure to treat the patient will have no untoward effect, as this is a self-limiting infection
d. Perform a dark-field examination of the lesion
e. Prescribe acyclovir for primary genital herpes

**195.** The laboratory reports that the Venereal Disease Research Laboratory (VDRL) test performed on the above patient is reactive at a dilution of 1:4 (4 dils). The patient also reports to you that he has recently been diagnosed with hepatitis A. Which one of the following is most appropriate next step in management?

a. Order a confirmatory test such as the fluorescent treponemal antibody (FTA) test
b. Order a rapid plasma reagin (RPR) test
c. Perform a spinal tap to rule out central nervous system (CNS) syphilis
d. Repeat the VDRL test
e. Report this patient to the health department, as he has syphilis

**196.** In the same patient, which of the following test combinations for syphilis is most appropriate?

a. FTA-Abs (IgG)/FTA-Abs (IgM)
b. RPR/culture of the lesion
c. RPR/FTA-Abs
d. *T. pallidum* hemagglutination (TPHA)/microhemagglutination—*T. pallidum* (MHTP) tests
e. VDRL/RPR

**197.** Assume that the patient absolutely denies any contact, sexual or otherwise, with a person who had syphilis. Assume also that both the RPR and the FTA-Abs are positive on this patient. Which of the following tests could be used to show that this patient probably does not have syphilis?

a. Frei test
b. MHTP test
c. Quantitative RPR
d. *Treponema pallidum* immobilization (TPI) test
e. VDRL

**198.** A 55-year-old man who is being treated for adenocarcinoma of the lung is admitted to a hospital because of a temperature of 38.9°C (102°F), chest pain, and a dry cough. Sputum is collected. Gram stain of the sputum is unremarkable, and culture reveals many small, gram-negative rods able to grow only on a charcoal yeast extract agar. Which of the following is the most likely organism?

a. Chlamydia trachomatis
b. Klebsiella pneumoniae
c. Legionella pneumophila
d. M. pneumoniae
e. S. aureus

**199.** A patient was hospitalized after an automobile accident. The wounds became infected, and the patient was treated with tobramycin, carbenicillin, and clindamycin. Five days after antibiotic therapy was initiated, the patient developed severe diarrhea and pseudomembranous enterocolitis. Antibiotic-associated diarrhea and the more serious pseudomembranous enterocolitis can be caused by which of the following organisms?

a. B. fragilis
b. Clostridium difficile
c. Clostridium perfringens
d. Clostridium sordellii
e. S. aureus

**200.** A premature neonate suffers pneumonia and sepsis. Sputum culture on blood agar plate yields pin-pointed β-hemolytic colonies. Which of the following is a simple test to determine whether the organism is *Streptococcus agalactiae* or *L. monocytogenes* (these two organisms are important neonatal pathogens)?

a. Bacitracin sensitivity test
b. Catalase test
c. Coagulase test
d. Polymerase chain reaction (PCR)
e. Sugar fermentation test

**201.** A 2-year-old child has a high fever and is irritable. He has a stiff neck. Gram stain smear of spinal fluid reveals gram-negative, small pleomorphic coccobacillary organisms. What is the most appropriate procedure to follow in order to reach an etiological diagnosis?

a. Culture the spinal fluid in chocolate agar, and identify the organism by growth factors
b. Culture the spinal fluid in mannitol-salt agar
c. Perform a catalase test of the isolated organism
d. Perform a coagulase test with the isolate
e. Perform a latex agglutination (LA) test to detect the specific antibody in the spinal fluid

**202.** A patient complains to his dentist about a draining lesion in his mouth. A Gram stain of the pus shows a few gram-positive cocci, leukocytes, and many-branched gram-positive rods. Branched yellow sulfur granules are observed by microscopy. Which of the following is the most likely cause of the disease?

a. *Actinomyces israelii*
b. *Actinomyces viscosus*
c. *C. diphtheriae*
d. *Propionibacterium acnes*
e. *S. aureus*

**203.** A female infant was born prematurely after rupture of membranes and, within 1 day of birth, developed a fever and died. The pregnant mother had been cultured just prior to the birth of her child, and her vaginal culture revealed group B streptococci (*S. agalactiae*). Which of the tests shown in the following figure would provide the most rapid and useful information?

a. A
b. B
c. C
d. D

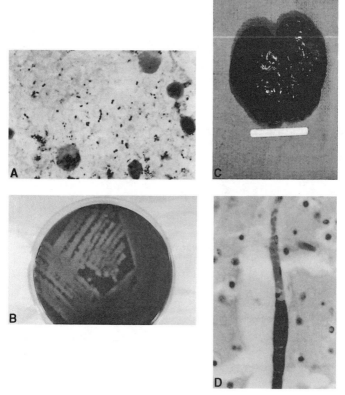

**A.** Direct Gram stain demonstrating *Streptococcus agalactiae* in CSF of infected neonate (μ1000). **B.** Blood agar plate demonstrating diffuse β-hemolysis due to group B streptococci from CSF. **C.** Brain at autopsy demonstrating acute hemorrhagic response to *S. agalactiae*. **D.** Brain section with blood vessel occluded by group B streptococci.

**204.** A 39-year-old primigravid Causian female lawyer develops premature rupture of the membrane at 35 weeks of gestation. She develops fever up to 103°F, and the amniotic fluid reveals group B *Streptococcus*. Which of the following is the best option to reduce Group B streptococcal infection in her fetus?

a. Identification of possible high-risk births
b. Intravenous penicillin administered at least 4 hours before delivery
c. Screening of pregnant females at the first office visit, usually during the first trimester
d. Screening of pregnant females in the last trimester
e. Use of a polysaccharide vaccine

**205.** A 1-week-old neonate presents to the pediatric emergency room with fever, irritability, poor feeding, and a bulging anterior fontanelle. Lumbar puncture is performed, and the cerebrospinal fluid (CSF) grows group B *Streptococcus*. Which of the following is the most likely pathogenic mechanism?

a. Complement C5a, a potent chemoattractant, activates polymorphonuclear neutrophils (PMNs)
b. In the absence of a specific antibody, opsonization, phagocyte recognition, and killing do not proceed normally
c. The alternative complement pathway is activated
d. The streptococci are resistant to penicillin

**206.** A man who has a penile chancre appears in a hospital's emergency service. The VDRL test is negative. Which of the following is the most appropriate course of action?

a. Perform dark-field microscopy for treponemes
b. Perform a Gram stain on the chancre fluid
c. Repeat the VDRL test in 10 days
d. Send the patient home untreated
e. Swab the chancre and culture on Thayer-Martin agar

**207.** A clinically depressed farmer complains of great weakness, a daily rise and fall in fever, and night sweats. Small gram-negative rods are isolated from blood cultures after 2 weeks' incubation. Which of the following organisms is the most likely etiologic agent?

a. *Brucella melitensis*
b. *C. jejuni*
c. *Francisella tularensis*
d. *S. enteritidis*
e. *Serratia marcescens*

**208.** An outbreak occurred in a community where the water supply was contaminated. Multiple patients experienced nausea and vomiting, as well as profuse diarrhea with abdominal cramps. Stools were described as "rice water." Curved, gram-negative rods were isolated on this sulfate-citrate-bile-sucrose agar. In the treatment of patients who have cholera, the use of a drug that inhibits adenyl cyclase would be expected to have which of the following characteristics?

a. Block the action of cholera toxin
b. Eradicate the organism
c. Increase fluid secretion
d. Kill the patient immediately
e. Reduce intestinal motility

**209.** A box of ham sandwiches with mayonnaise, prepared by a person with a boil on his neck, was left out of the refrigerator for the on-call interns. Three doctors became violently ill approximately 2 hours after eating the sandwiches. Which of the following is the most likely cause?

a. *C. perfringens* toxin
b. Coagulase from *S. aureus* in the ham
c. Penicillinase given to inactivate penicillin in the pork
d. *S. aureus* enterotoxin
e. *S. aureus* leukocidin

**210.** A 34-year-old diabetic truck driver notices maceration of the web space of his toes on the right foot. Two days later he has a temperature of up to 100°F, exquisite tenderness, erythema, and swelling of the right leg. Culture exudate from the foot yields *S. aureus*. Which of the following often complicates treatment of *S. aureus* infection with penicillin?

a. Allergic reaction caused by staphylococcal protein
b. Inability of penicillin to penetrate the membrane of *S. aureus*
c. Lack of penicillin binding sites on *S. aureus*
d. Production of penicillin acetylase by *S. aureus*
e. Production of penicillinase by *S. aureus*

**211.** Two of three family members had dinner at a local restaurant and, within 48 hours, experienced double vision, difficulty in swallowing and speaking, and breathing problems. These symptoms are consistent with which of the following?

a. Activation of cyclic AMP
b. Endotoxin shock
c. Ingestion of a neurotoxin
d. Invasion of the gut epithelium by an organism
e. Secretion of an enterotoxin

**212.** Several *Neisseria* species are a part of the normal flora (commensals) of the human upper respiratory tract. Which of the following statements accurately describes the significance of these bacteria?

a. As a part of the normal flora, Neisseriae provide a natural immunity in local host defense
b. As a part of the respiratory flora, they are the most common cause of acute bronchitis and pneumonia
c. Commensal bacteria stimulate a cell-mediated immunity (CMI)
d. Commensal Neisseriae in the upper respiratory tract impede phagocytosis by means of lipoteichoic acid
e. Normal flora such as nonpathogenic Neisseriae provide effective nonspecific B-cell-mediated humoral immunity

**213.** A family routinely consumed unpasteurized milk, claiming "better taste." Several members experienced a sudden onset of crampy abdominal pain, fever, and bloody, profuse diarrhea. *C. jejuni* was isolated and identified from all patients. Which of the following is the treatment of choice for this type of enterocolitis?

a. Ampicillin
b. *Campylobacter* antitoxin
c. Ciprofloxacin
d. Erythromycin
e. Pepto-Bismol

**214.** An unimmunized 2-year-old boy presents with drooling from the mouth, elevated temperature, and enlarged tonsils. During attempts at intubation, no grey-white membrane is observed but the epiglottis appears "beefy" red and edematous. Which of the following is the most likely organism?

a. *Haemophilus hemolyticus*
b. *H. influenzae*
c. *K. pneumoniae*
d. *M. pneumoniae*
e. *Neisseria meningitidis*

### Item 215–217

A 70-year-old female patient is re-admitted to a local hospital with fever and chills following cardiac surgery at a major teaching institution. A gram-positive coccus grows within 24 hours from blood taken from the patient. Initial tests indicated that this isolate is resistant to penicillin.

**215.** Which of the following is the most likely identification?

a. *Enterococcus*
b. Group A *Streptococcus*
c. Group B *Streptococcus*
d. *Neisseria* species
e. *S. pneumoniae*

**216.** Further testing reveals that the isolate possesses the group D antigen, and is not β-lactamase-positive, but is resistant to vancomycin. Which of the following is the most likely identification of this isolate?

a. *Enterococcus cassiflavus*
b. *Enterococcus durans*
c. *Enterococcus faecalis*
d. *Enterococcus faecium*
e. *S. pneumoniae*

**217.** Which of the following is the treatment of choice for the isolate in question 216?

a. Ciprofloxacin
b. Gentamicin
c. Gentamicin and ampicillin
d. Rifampin
e. No available treatment

**218.** Acute hematogenous osteomyelitis is often diagnosed by isolation of the organism from the blood and is caused most often by which of the following organisms?

a. *E. coli*
b. *Proteus mirabilis*
c. *S. aureus*
d. *Staphylococcus epidermidis*
e. *Streptococcus faecalis*

**219.** A 3-year-old girl, with no history of vaccination, is brought to the hospital with a sore throat, fever, malaise, and difficulty breathing. Physical examination reveals a gray membrane covering the pharynx. Growth of the etiologic agent on cysteine-tellurite agar forms gray to black colonies with a brown halo. The major virulence factor of this organism is only produced by those strains that will most likely have which of the following characteristics?

a. Encapsulated
b. Glucose fermenters
c. Lysogenic for β-prophage
d. Of the mitis strain
e. Sucrose fermenters

### Item 220–222

A 28-year-old menstruating woman appears in the emergency room with the following signs and symptoms: fever, 104°F (40°C); WBC, 16,000/µL; blood pressure, 90/65 mmHg; a scarlatiniform rash on her trunk, palms, and soles; extreme fatigue; vomiting; and diarrhea.

**220.** Which of the following is the most likely diagnosis?
a. Chickenpox
b. Guillain-Barré syndrome
c. Scalded skin syndrome
d. Staphylococcal food poisoning
e. Toxic shock syndrome (TSS)

**221.** Culture of the menstrual fluid in this case cited would most likely reveal a predominance of which of the following?
a. *C. difficile*
b. *C. perfringens*
c. *Gardnerilla vaginalis*
d. *S. aureus*
e. *No organisms isolated*

**222.** Which of the following is the most characteristic finding not yet revealed in the case just presented?
a. A meal of chicken in a fast-food restaurant
b. A retained tampon
c. Heavy menstrual flow
d. Recent exposure to rubella
e. Travel to Vermont

### Item 223–224

A new LA reagent for *H. influenzae* polysaccharide antigen in CSF was evaluated. Results were compared with the isolation of *H. influenzae* from the CSF. Results were as follows:

LA POS, CULT POS: 25
LA POS, CULT NEG: 5
LA NEG, CULT POS: 5
LA NEG, CULT NEG: 95

**223.** Which of the following best indicates the sensitivity of LA?

a. 0%
b. 30%
c. 85%
d. 95%
e. 100%

**224.** Which of the following best indicates the specificity of LA?

a. 0%
b. 30%
c. 80%
d. 95%
e. 100%

**225.** A severely burned firefighter develops a rapidly disseminating bacterial infection while hospitalized. "Green pus" is noted in the burned tissue, and cultures of both the tissue and blood yield small, oxidase-positive, gram-negative rods. Which of the following statements about this organism is correct?

a. Endotoxin is the only virulence factor known to be produced by these bacteria
b. Humans are the only known reservoir hosts for these bacteria
c. The bacteria are difficult to culture because they have numerous growth requirements
d. These are among the most antibiotic resistant of all clinically relevant bacteria
e. These highly motile bacteria can "swarm" over the surface of culture media

**226.** Several hours after dining on sweet and sour chicken and pork fried rice at the home of an Asian friend, a 34-year-old car salesman exhibits abdominal discomfort, nausea, and vomiting. In the middle of the night he awakens with watery diarrhea. Which of the following pairs of organisms is routinely responsible for food poisoning?

a. *Clostridium botulinum* and *Bacillus anthracis*
b. *C. difficile* and *C. botulinum*
c. *C. perfringens* and *Bacillus cereus*
d. *C. tetani* and *B. anthracis*
e. *Clostridium t.* and *B. cereus*

**227.** MRSA was isolated from seven patients in a 14-bed intensive care unit. All patients were isolated and the unit closed to any more admissions. Which of the following best explains these rigorous methods to control MRSA?

a. MRSA causes TSS
b. MRSA is inherently more virulent than other staphylococci
c. MRSA is resistant to penicillin
d. MRSA spreads more rapidly from patient to patient than antibiotic-susceptible staphylococci do
e. The alternative for treatment of MRSA is vancomycin, an expensive and potentially toxic antibiotic

**228.** A patient with AIDS returns from Haiti with acute diarrhea. The stool reveals an oval organism (8–9 μm in diameter) that is acid-fast and fluoresces blue under ultraviolet light. The most likely identification of this organism is which of the following?

a. *Cryptosporidium*
b. *Cyclospora*
c. *Enterocytozoon*
d. *Giardia*
e. *Prototheca*

**229.** A 2-year-old infant is brought to the emergency room with hematuria, fever, and thrombocytopenia. Which one of the following bacteria would most likely be isolated from a stool specimen?

a. *Aeromonas* species
b. *Enterobacter aerogenes*
c. *E. coli* 0157/H7
d. *S. enteriditis*
e. *Shigella flexneri*

**230.** A 65-year-old healthy retired former executive female went on her yearly vacation to Mexico. Unlike her previous trips she decided to use the local water to make her favorite punch. Thirty-six hours later she developed profused watery diarrhea, severe cramping, and abdominal pain. She was diagnosed with *E. coli* related diarrhea. Which of the following *E. coli* types is characterized by the presence of heat-labile (LT) and heat-stable (ST) proteins?

a. Enteroinvasive (EIEC)
b. Enterotoxigenic (ETEC)
c. Enterohemorrhagic (EHEC)
d. Enteropathogenic (EPEC)
e. Enterohemolytic (EHEEC)

**231.** A 48-year-old farmer in New Mexico is bitten by a flea and, 5 days later, develops a sudden onset of fever, chills, weakness, and headache. A few hours later he develops buboes in the right axilla and groin which are intensely painful. This patient is subsequently diagnosed with bubonic plague and does not develop any pneumonic features of the disease. Human plague can be bubonic or pneumonic. Which of the following is the primary epidemiologic difference between the two clinical forms of plague?

a. Age of the patient
b. Geographic location of the animal vector
c. Health of the animal vector
d. Route of infection
e. Season of the year

**232.** A 9-year-old child is brought to the emergency room with the chief complaint of enlarged, painful axillary lymph nodes. The resident physician also notes a small, inflamed, dime-sized lesion surrounding what appears to be a small scratch on the forearm. The lymph node is aspirated and some pus is sent to the laboratory for examination. A Warthin-Starry silver impregnation stain reveals many highly pleomorphic, rod-shaped bacteria. Which of the following is the most likely cause of this infection?

a. *Bartonella henselae*
b. *Brucella canis*
c. *Mycobacterium scrofulaceum*
d. *Y. enterocolitica*
e. *Yersinia pestis*

**233.** A sixth-grade boy returned from summer camp with several minor cuts and abrasions. Within a week, extensive cellulitis developed, and it was apparent that subcutaneous tissue was involved, requiring surgical intervention of nonviable tissue. Antibiotics were used aggressively. This is usually caused by which of the following?

a. *B. cereus*
b. *C. tetani*
c. Group A streptococci
d. *Micrococcus species*
e. *S. aureus*

**234.** A 40-year-old female reports chronic gastritis. She tests positive for *H. pylori*. After a course of the appropiate antibiotic theraphy her symptoms subside. Which of the following is the most effective noninvasive test for the diagnosis of *Helicobacter*-associated gastric ulcers?

a. Culture of stomach contents for *H. pylori*
b. Detection of *H. pylori* antigen in stool
c. Growth of *H. pylori* from a stomach biopsy
d. Growth of *H. pylori* in the stool
e. IgM antibodies to *H. pylori*

**235.** The following test results were observed in a woman tested in November who reported being in the woods in Pennsylvania during the past summer, was bitten by a tick, and now has a flattened red area near the bite with central clearing. She also had flulike illness with fever, myalgia, and headache. Which of the following is the most appropriate course of action?

a. Ask the patient if she has a severe headache
b. Do a spinal tap for CSF
c. Observe the lesion
d. Order a Lyme disease antibody titer
e. Start treatment with tetracycline

**236.** *Mycobacterium avium* is a major opportunistic pathogen in AIDS patients. *M. avium* from AIDS patients is best characterized by which one of the following statements?

a. Few isolates from AIDS patients are acid-fast
b. Most isolates from AIDS patients are sensitive to isoniazid and streptomycin
c. *M. avium* can be isolated from the blood of many AIDS patients
d. *M. avium* isolates from AIDS patients are of multiple serovars
e. The majority of *M. avium* isolates from AIDS patients are nonpigmented

**237.** A 12-year old girl experienced a GAS pharyngitis and within 3 weeks had chest pain and developed new murmurs of mitral regurgitation. Which of the following statements best typifies the disease she experienced?

a. It is a complication of group A streptococcal skin disease but usually not of pharyngitis
b. It is characterized by inflammatory lesions that may involve the heart, joints, subcutaneous tissues, and CNS
c. It is very common in developing countries but extremely rare and decreasing in incidence in the United States
d. Prophylaxis with benzathine penicillin is of little value
e. The pathogenesis is related to the similarity between a staphylococcal antigen and a human cardiac antigen

**238.** After extraction of a wisdom tooth, an 18-year-old male student is diagnosed with subacute bacterial endocarditis. He has a congenital heart disease that has been under control. Which of the following is the most likely organism causing his infection?

a.  S. aureus
b.  S. epidermidis
c.  S. pneumoniae
d.  Streptococcus viridians
e.  E. faecalis

**239.** A 64-year-old sheepherder from the farming region of central California is rushed to the emergency room in anaphylactic shock. The history, as told by the ambulance medic, is that the man was hit in the abdomen during a bar-room brawl. Ultrasound reveals a large cyst mass in the liver. A cautious needle aspiration of the liver mass reveals "hydatid sand." Which of the following is the most likely agent involved?

a.  Ascaris
b.  Clonorchis
c.  Echinococcus
d.  Fasciolopsis
e.  Schistosoma

**240.** A 70-year-old male is taken to the emergency room with a history of "cold-like" symptoms for at least 3 days. At the time of the visit, his temperature is 102°F and he experienced shaking, chills, chest pain, and a productive cough with bloody sputum. Blood agar culture reveals gram-positive α-hemolytic colonies. If a quellung test was done on the colonies, which of the following bacteria would most likely be positive?

a.  C. diphtheriae
b.  Enterobacter
c.  Haemophilus parainfluenzae
d.  Neisseria gonorrhoeae
e.  S. pneumoniae

**241.** A 6-month old infant is admitted to the hospital with acute meningitis. The Gram stain reveals gram-positive, short rods, and the mother indicates that the child has received "all" of the meningitis vaccinations. Which of the following is the most likely cause of the disease?

a. *H. influenzae*
b. *L. monocytogenes*
c. *N. meningitidis*, group A
d. *N. meningitidis*, group C
e. *S. pneumoniae*

**242.** A 40-year old man presents to the emergency medicine department 1 week following a foot injury. He is experiencing intense pain in the area of injury and the muscles of the jaw. Which of the following is the most common portal of entry for the etiologic organism?

a. Gastrointestinal tract
b. Genital tract
c. Nasal tract
d. Respiratory tract
e. Skin

**243.** A 22-year-old homeless person with a known drug abuse problem and multiple opportunistic infections tests positive in a PPD-S test. Which of the following is the most common way this infection is acquired?

a. Gastrointestinal tract
b. Genital tract
c. Nasal tract
d. Respiratory tract
e. Skin

**244.** A 31-year-old school teacher returns from foreign travel and experiences a sudden (1–2 days) onset of abdominal pain, fever, and watery diarrhea, caused by a heat-labile exotoxin that affects both the gut and the CNS. This infection is caused by an etiologic agent commonly acquired through which of the following routes?

a. Gastrointestinal tract
b. Genital tract
c. Nasal tract
d. Respiratory tract
e. Skin

**245.** A college student was surprised one morning by painful urination and a creamy-colored exudate. Any person who acquires the gram-negative microbe that causes this infection is most likely to have acquired it via which of the following?

a. Gastrointestinal tract
b. Genitourinary tract
c. Nasal tract
d. Respiratory tract
e. Skin

**246.** A 25-year-old college student with no history of allergic rhinitis has a 12-day history of facial pain, clear rhinorrhea, fever, headache, and back pain. Her symptoms did not respond to over-the-counter medication. Culture of the fluid from the sinus reveals *Moraxella (Branhamella) catarrhalis*. Which of the following statements best characterizes *M. catarrhalis*?

a. A gram-negative, pleomorphic rod that can cause endocarditis
b. A gram-negative rod, fusiform-shaped, that is associated with periodontal disease but may cause sepsis
c. The causative agent of rat-bite fever
d. The causative agent of sinusitis, bronchitis, and pneumonia
e. The causative agent of trench fever

**247.** A 16-year-old Hispanic female with poor oral hygiene and severe gingivitis presents with a temperature of 103.5°F and hypotension. Blood culture is positive for *Capnocytophaga*. Which of the following statements best characterizes *Capnocytophaga*?

a. A gram-negative, pleomorphic rod that can cause endocarditis
b. A gram-negative rod, fusiform-shaped, that is associated with periodontal disease but may cause sepsis
c. The causative agent of rat-bite fever
d. The causative agent of sinusitis, bronchitis, and pneumonia
e. The causative agent of trench fever

**248.** Several employees in a veterinary facility experienced a mild influenza-like infection after working on six sheep with an undiagnosed illness. The etiologic agent causing the human disease is most often transmitted to humans by which of the following methods?

a. Fecal contamination from flea deposits on the skin
b. Inhalation of infected aerosols from animal urine and feces
c. Lice feces scratched into the broken skin during the louse's blood feeding
d. Tick saliva during feeding on human blood
e. Urethral discharge from infected humans

**249.** An enterococcus (*E. faecium*) is isolated from a urine specimen (100,000 cfu/mL). Treatment of the patient with ampicillin and gentamicin fails. Which of the following is the most clinically appropriate action?

a. Consider vancomycin as an alternative drug
b. Determine if fluorescent microscopy is available for the diagnosis of actinomycosis
c. Do no further clinical workup
d. Suggest to the laboratory that low colony counts may reflect infection
e. Suggest a repeat antibiotic susceptibility test

**250.** A patient with symptoms of a urinary tract infection had a culture taken, which grew $5 \times 10^3$ *E. coli*. The laboratory reported it as "insignificant." Which of the following is the most appropriate step in management?

a. Consider vancomycin as an alternative drug
b. Determine if fluorescent microscopy is available for the diagnosis of actinomycosis
c. Do no further clinical workup
d. Suggest to the laboratory that low colony counts may reflect infection
e. Suggest a repeat antibiotic susceptibility test

**251.** A patient appears in the emergency room with a submandibular mass. A smear is made of the drainage and a bewildering variety of bacteria are seen, including branched, gram-positive rods. Which of the following is the most clinically appropriate action?

a. Consider vancomycin as an alternative drug
b. Determine if fluorescent microscopy is available for the diagnosis of actinomycosis
c. Do no further clinical workup
d. Suggest to the laboratory that low colony counts may reflect infection
e. Suggest a repeat antibiotic susceptibility test

**252.** A 55-year-old male develops malaise, fever up to 103.5°C, non-productive cough, headache, and shortness of breath, a few days after he repaired the cooling system of an old hotel. A chest x-ray reveals fluid in his lungs. From a sputum sample, a gram-negative rod grew slowly on a buffered cysteine containing charcoal-yeast agar. Which of the following antibiotic therapies is most appropiate for treating this patient?

a. Ampicillin
b. Ceftriaxone
c. Erythromycin
d. Penicillin
e. Vancomycin

**253.** A 60-year-old male resident from a nursing home presents to the emergency room with a fever of 41°C, shaking chills, severe pain to the right side of his chest that worsens with breathing, and a productive cough with blood-tinged sputum. During the previous 3 days, he noted cold-like symptoms. Gram stain evaluation of the sputum reveals gram-positive diplococci that grow into α-hemolytic colonies on blood agar. Which of the following antibiotic therapies is the most appropiate treatment for this patient?

a. Ampicillin
b. Ceftriaxone
c. Erythromycin
d. Penicillin
e. Vancomycin

**254.** A 12-year-old boy, after a camping trip near a wooded area in Northern California, is taken to the emergency room after complaining of a headache. He has an erythema migrans rash around what appears to be a tick bite. Which of the following is the antibiotic of choice for treating this patient?

a. Ampicillin
b. Ceftriaxone
c. Erythromycin
d. Penicillin
e. Vancomycin

**255.** A 6-year-old girl presents to her pediatrician with fever, headache, and a sore throat. She has swollen tender cervical lymph nodes, and her oropharynx is red with a gray-white exudate covering both her tonsils. A rapid strep test of her throat swab is positive, and the culture subsequently grows β-hemolytic *Streptococcus*. Which of the following antibiotic therapies is most appropiate for treating this patient?

a. Ampicillin
b. Ceftriaxone
c. Erythromycin
d. Penicillin
e. Vancomycin

**256.** A young woman being treated with a broad-spectrum antimicrobial develops endoscopically observed microabscesses and diarrhea. Which of the following is the therapy of choice for this form of enterocolitis?

a. Ampicillin
b. Ceftriaxone
c. Erythromycin
d. Penicillin
e. Vancomycin

**257.** Although cholera, a *Vibrio* infection, has rarely been seen in the United States, there have been recent outbreaks of classic cholera associated with shellfish harvested from the Gulf of Mexico. Vibrios are shaped like curved rods, and infections more common than cholera may be caused by a variety of curved-rod bacteria. Which of the following best describes *C. jejuni*?

a. Cause of gastroenteritis; reservoir in birds and mammals, optimal growth at 42°C
b. Human pathogen, halophilic, lactose-negative, sucrose-negative; causes gastrointestinal diseases primarily from ingestion of under-cooked seafood
c. Human pathogen, halophilic, lactose-positive; produces heat-labile, extracellular toxin
d. "String-test"—positive isolate; three serotypes—Ogawa (AB), Inaba (AC), Hikojima (ABC)
e. Urease-positive; cause of fetal distress in cattle

**258.** V. *cholerae*, the causative agent of cholera, is best described by which of the following statements?

a. Cause of gastroenteritis; reservoir in birds and mammals, optimal growth at 42°C
b. Human pathogen, halophilic, lactose-negative, sucrose-negative; causes gastrointestinal diseases primarily from ingestion of under-cooked seafood
c. Human pathogen, halophilic, lactose-positive; produces heat-labile, extracellular toxin
d. "String-test"—positive isolate; three serotypes—Ogawa (AB), Inaba (AC), Hikojima (ABC)
e. Urease-positive; cause of fetal distress in cattle

**259.** A 20-year-old female in post-Katerina New Orleans eats poorly cooked seafood (oysters, clams, and mollusks) for her birthday dinner. Twenty-four hours later, she develops explosive watery diarrhea and abdominal cramps. She is positive for V. *parahaemolyticus*. Which of the following statements best describes this organism?

a. Cause of gastroenteritis; reservoir in birds and mammals, optimal growth at 42° C
b. Human pathogen, halophilic, lactose-negative, sucrose-negative; causes gastrointestinal diseases primarily from ingestion of under-cooked seafood
c. Human pathogen, halophilic, lactose-positive; produces heat-labile, extracellular toxin
d. "String-test"—positive isolate; three serotypes—Ogawa (AB), Inaba (AC), Hikojima (ABC)
e. Urease-positive; cause of fetal distress in cattle

**260.** A 25-year-old male was wading through brackish water in post-Katerina New Orleans. He has a history of hepatitis C. He develops worsening abdominal pain and jaundice. Regarding *Vibrio vulnificus*, which of the following statements best describes this organism?

a. Cause of gastroenteritis; reservoir in birds and mammals, optimal growth at 42°C
b. Human pathogen, halophilic, lactose-negative, sucrose-negative; causes gastrointestinal diseases primarily from ingestion of under-cooked seafood
c. Human pathogen, halophilic, lactose-positive; produces heat-labile, extracellular toxin
d. "String-test"—positive isolate; three serotypes—Ogawa (AB), Inaba (AC), Hikojima (ABC)
e. Urease-positive; cause of fetal distress in cattle

**261.** *Y. enterocolitica,* formerly a *Pasteurella,* is best described by which of the following statements?

a. Commonly inhabits the canine respiratory tract and is an occasional pathogen for humans; strongly urease-positive
b. Manifests different biochemical and physiologic characteristics, depending on growth temperature, and causes a spectrum of human disease, most commonly mesenteric lymphadenitis
c. Pits agar, grows both in carbon dioxide and under anaerobic conditions, and is part of the normal oral cavity flora
d. Typically infects cattle, requires 5–10% carbon dioxide for growth, and is inhibited by the dye thionine
e. Typically is found in infected animal bites in humans and can cause hemorrhagic septicemia in animals

**262.** *B. abortus,* one of the three species causing brucellosis, a possible bioterrorism agent, is best described by which of the following statements?

a. Commonly inhabits the canine respiratory tract and is an occasional pathogen for humans; strongly urease-positive
b. Manifests different biochemical and physiologic characteristics, depending on growth temperature, and causes a spectrum of human disease, most commonly mesenteric lymphadenitis
c. Pits agar, grows both in carbon dioxide and under anaerobic conditions, and is part of the normal oral cavity flora
d. Typically infects cattle, requires 5–10% carbon dioxide for growth, and is inhibited by the dye thionine
e. Typically is found in infected animal bites in humans and can cause hemorrhagic septicemia in animals

**263.** *Bordetella bronchiseptica* could be confused with the agent of whooping cough. It is best described by which of the following statements?

a. Commonly inhabits the canine respiratory tract and is an occasional pathogen for humans; strongly urease-positive
b. Manifests different biochemical and physiologic characteristics, depending on growth temperature, and causes a spectrum of human disease, most commonly mesenteric lymphadenitis
c. Pits agar, grows both in carbon dioxide and under anaerobic conditions, and is part of the normal oral cavity flora
d. Typically infects cattle, requires 5–10% carbon dioxide for growth, and is inhibited by the dye thionine
e. Typically is found in infected animal bites in humans and can cause hemorrhagic septicemia in animals

**264.** *P. multocida* is a very common organism and is best described by which of the following statements?

a.  Commonly inhabits the canine respiratory tract and is an occasional pathogen for humans; strongly urease-positive
b.  Manifests different biochemical and physiologic characteristics, depending on growth temperature, and causes a spectrum of human disease, most commonly mesenteric lymphadenitis
c.  Pits agar, grows both in carbon dioxide and under anaerobic conditions, and is part of the normal oral cavity flora
d.  Typically infects cattle, requires 5–10% carbon dioxide for growth, and is inhibited by the dye thionine
e.  Typically is found in infected animal bites in humans and can cause hemorrhagic septicemia in animals

**265.** A 26-year-old male presents to his family physician with complaints of painful burning during urination and a milky discharge. The purulent discharge revealed many neutrophils with intracellular gram-negative diplococci. Which of the following mediums would most likely be used for isolating *N. gonorrhoeae*, the suspected organism?

a.  Löffler's medium
b.  Löwenstein-Jensen medium
c.  Sheep blood agar
d.  Thayer-Martin agar
e.  Thiosulfate citrate bile salts sucrose medium

**266.** Twenty-four hours after returning from a short trip to Asia, a 35-year-old female has a sudden onset of vomiting and massive watery diarrhea that is colorless, odorless, and contains flecks of mucus. Which of the following mediums would most likely be used for isolating *V. cholerae*, the suspected organism?

a.  Löffler's medium
b.  Löwenstein-Jensen medium
c.  Sheep blood agar
d.  Thayer-Martin agar
e.  Thiosulfate citrate bile salts sucrose medium

**267.** A 32-year-old female prostitute is seen at the public health clinic with fever, night sweats, and coughing blood. History reveals she is HIV positive and has lost 20 pounds over the past month. Acid-fast bacilli are observed in the sputum. After digestion of the sputum, isolation of the suspected organism is best accomplished by using which one of the following media?

a. Löffler's medium
b. Löwenstein-Jensen medium
c. Sheep blood agar
d. Thayer-Martin agar
e. Thiosulfate citrate bile salts sucrose medium

**268.** Antibiotic therapy may be a critical step in the management of patients infected with the following microorganisms. Which organism listed below would not benefit from prompt antibiotic treatment?

a. *B. anthracis*
b. *C. botulinum*
c. *C. difficile*
d. *C. perfringens*
e. *C. tetani*

**269.** A 12-year-old boy has sudden onset of fever, headache, and stiff neck. Two days earlier, he swam in a lake that is believed to have been contaminated with dog excreta. Leptospirosis is suspected. Which of the following laboratory tests is most appropriate to determine whether he has been infected with leptospira?

a. Agglutination test for leptospiral antigen
b. Counterimmunoelectrophoresis of urine sample
c. Gram stain of urine specimen
d. Spinal fluid for dark-field microscopy and culture in Fletcher's serum medium
e. Urine culture on EMB and Thayer-Martin agar

**270.** A 60-year-old female complains of tenderness and pain around a peritoneal catheter. Blood cultures reveal gram-positive, catalase-positive cocci. Which of the following is the most likely organism which is also considered a predominant organism on skin?

a.  α-hemolytic streptococci
b.  *B. fragilis*
c.  *E. coli*
d.  *Lactobacillus*
e.  *S. epidermidis*

**271.** A healthy 45-year-old female had root canal treatment about 3 weeks ago. She now presents with a new heart murmur, fever, painful skin nodules, and abdominal pain, with an abnormal liver function test. Which of the following organisms would mostly likely cause endocarditis and be implicated in dental caries or root canal infections?

a.  α-Hemolytic Streptococci
b.  *B. fragilis*
c.  *E. coli*
d.  *Lactobacillus*
e.  *S. epidermidis*

**272.** A 17-year-old man is hospitalized with trauma to the abdomen following a gang-related fight. He develops an intra-abdominal abscess which is drained and sent to the laboratory. A mixture of gram-negative anaerobes are detected. Which of the following microorganisms is the most likely and is also the most prevalent bacterium in the gut?

a.  α-Hemolytic Streptococci
b.  *B. fragilis*
c.  *E. coli*
d.  *Lactobacillus*
e.  *S. epidermidis*

**273.** A 25-year-old female is treated with a course of broad-spectrum antibiotics for severe pelvic inflammatory disease. She now reports a thick milky white pruritic vaginal discharge. Which of the following is the most prevalent microorganism in the vagina and may also be protective?

a. α-Hemolytic Streptococci
b. *B. fragilis*
c. *E. coli*
d. *Lactobacillus*
e. *S. epidermidis*

**274.** *Streptococcus mutans* is best described by which of the following statements?

a. An anaerobic, filamentous bacterium that often causes cervicofacial osteomyelitis
b. A β-hemolytic organism that causes a diffuse, rapidly spreading cellulitis
c. A facultative anaerobe that is highly cariogenic and sticks to teeth by synthesis of a dextran
d. A facultative anaerobe that often inhabits the buccal mucosa early in a neonate's life and can cause bacterial endocarditis
e. A facultatively anaerobic, rod-shaped bacterium that sticks to teeth and is cariogenic

**275.** *Streptococcus salivarius,* a common isolate in the clinical laboratory, is best described by which of the following statements?

a. An anaerobic, filamentous bacterium that often causes cervicofacial osteomyelitis
b. A β-hemolytic organism that causes a diffuse, rapidly spreading cellulitis
c. A facultative anaerobe that is highly cariogenic and sticks to teeth by synthesis of a dextran
d. A facultative anaerobe that often inhabits the buccal mucosa early in a neonate's life and can cause bacterial endocarditis
e. A facultatively anaerobic, rod-shaped bacterium that sticks to teeth and is cariogenic

**276.** A. *israelii* is one of many actinomycetes and is best described by which of the following statements?

a. An anaerobic, filamentous bacterium that often causes cervicofacial osteomyelitis
b. A β-hemolytic organism that causes a diffuse, rapidly spreading cellulitis
c. A facultative anaerobe that is highly cariogenic and sticks to teeth by synthesis of a dextran
d. A facultative anaerobe that often inhabits the buccal mucosa early in a neonate's life and can cause bacterial endocarditis
e. A facultatively anaerobic, rod-shaped bacterium that sticks to teeth and is cariogenic

**277.** A. *viscosus,* a ubiquitous actinomycete, is best described by which of the following statements?

a. An anaerobic, filamentous bacterium that often causes cervicofacial osteomyelitis
b. A β-hemolytic organism that causes a diffuse, rapidly spreading cellulitis
c. A facultative anaerobe that is highly cariogenic and sticks to teeth by synthesis of a dextran
d. A facultative anaerobe that often inhabits the buccal mucosa early in a neonate's life and can cause bacterial endocarditis
e. A facultatively anaerobic, rod-shaped bacterium that sticks to teeth and is cariogenic

**278.** A 3-year-old girl from a family that does not believe in immunization presents to the emergency room with a sore throat, fever, malaise, and difficulty breathing. A gray membrane covering the pharynx is observed on physical emamination. Which of the following best describes C. *diphtheriae,* the etiologic agent?

a. It produces at least one protein toxin consisting of two subunits, A and B, that cause severe spasmodic cough, usually in children
b. It produces a toxin that blocks protein synthesis in an infected cell and carries a lytic bacteriophage that produces the genetic information for toxin production
c. It secretes an erythrogenic toxin that causes the characteristic signs of scarlet fever
d. It secretes an exotoxin that has been called "verotoxin" and "Shiga-like toxin"; infection is mediated by specific attachment to mucosal membranes
e. It requires cysteine for growth

**279.** A 4-year-old boy is taken to see his pediatrician because of a persisi-tent cough that gradually worsened over a 12-day period. On the day of the examination the cough is so severe that it is frequently followed by vomit-ing. A blood cell count shows marked leukocytosis with a predominance of lymphocytes. Which of the following statements best characterizes this microorganism?

a. It produces a toxin that increases cAMP levels resulting in increased mucus production
b. It produces a toxin that blocks protein synthesis in an infected cell and carries a lytic bacteriophage that produces the genetic information for toxin production
c. It secretes an erythrogenic toxin that causes the characteristic signs of scarlet fever
d. It secretes an exotoxin that has been called "verotoxin" and "Shiga-like toxin"; infection is mediated by specific attachment to mucosal membranes
e. It requires cysteine for growth

**280.** A 48-year-old deer-hunter presents to the emergency room with lym-phadenopathy and a skin lesion which started as a painful papule at the site of a tick bite. The papule then ulcerates with a necrotic center and raised border. Asperate of the ulcer is positive for *F. tularensis*. Which one of the following statements best characterizes this bacterium?

a. It produces at least one protein toxin consisting of two subunits, A and B, that cause severe spasmodic cough, usually in children
b. It produces a toxin that blocks protein synthesis in an infected cell and carries a lytic bacteriophage that produces the genetic information for toxin production
c. It secretes an erythrogenic toxin that causes the characteristic signs of scarlet fever
d. It secretes an exotoxin that has been called "verotoxin" and "Shiga-like toxin"; infection is mediated by specific attachment to mucosal membranes
e. It requires cysteine for growth

**281.** Ten boy scouts are hospitalized with bloody diarrhea and severe hematological abnormalities. An investigation establishes that all of the boys developed symptoms following consumption of hamburgers from the same fast-food restaurant chain. Which of the following best describes *E. coli* 0157/H7, the etiologic bacterium responsible for the outbreak?

a.  It produces at least one protein toxin consisting of two subunits, A and B, that cause severe spasmodic cough, usually in children
b.  It produces a toxin that blocks protein synthesis in an infected cell and carries a lytic bacteriophage that produces the genetic information for toxin production
c.  It secretes an erythrogenic toxin that causes the characteristic signs of scarlet fever
d.  It secretes an exotoxin that has been called "verotoxin" and "Shiga-like toxin"; infection is mediated by specific attachment to mucosal membranes
e.  It requires cysteine for growth

**282.** A 4-year-old girl awakens at midnight complaining of a sore throat and headache, and she has a fever of 101°F. Physical examination reveals an erythematous throat. A rapid strep test is positive. A throat swab is sent to the laboratory for further testing. Which of the following statements best characterizes *Streptococcus pyogenes* as the presumed etiologic agent?

a.  It produces at least one protein toxin consisting of two subunits, A and B, that cause severe spasmodic cough, usually in children
b.  It produces a toxin that blocks protein synthesis in an infected cell and carries a lytic bacteriophage that produces the genetic information for toxin production
c.  It secretes an erythrogenic toxin that causes the characteristic signs of scarlet fever
d.  It secretes an exotoxin that has been called "verotoxin" and "Shiga-like toxin"; infection is mediated by specific attachment to mucosal membranes
e.  It has capsules of polyglutamic acid, which is toxic when injected into rabbits

**283.** A 19-year-old military recruit who lives in the barracks develops a macular papular skin rash, severe headache, photophobia, fever, stiff neck, and blurred vision. He is presumed to have *N. meningitidis*. Which of the following is a characteristic physiological trait of this organism?

a.  It causes spontaneous abortion and has tropism for placental tissue due to the presence of erythritol in allantoic and amniotic fluid
b.  It has a capsule of polyglutamic acid, which is toxic when injected into rabbits
c.  It possesses N-acetylneuraminic acid capsule and adheres to specific tissues by pili found on the bacterial cell surface
d.  It secretes two toxins, A and B, in the large bowel during antibiotic therapy
e.  It synthesizes protein toxin as a result of colonization of vaginal tampons

**284.** A 45-year-old cattle-farm worker goes to the public health clinic after experiencing 6 weeks of undulating fever, chills, sweating, headache, fatigue, muscle pain, and weight loss. History reveals that he enjoys drinking fresh unpasteurized milk with his other coworkers during the mid-morning breaks. A blood sample is sent to the state laboratory for serologic testing because the physician assistant suspects *Brucella* infection. Which of the following statements best characterizes this organism?

a. It causes spontaneous abortion and has tropism for placental tissue due to the presence of erythritol in allantoic and amniotic fluid
b. It has a capsule of polyglutamic acid, which is toxic when injected into rabbits
c. It has 82 polysaccharide capsular types; capsule is antiphagocytic; type 3 capsule (b-d-glucuronic acid polymer) most commonly seen in infected adults
d. It secretes two toxins, A and B, in the large bowel during antibiotic therapy
e. It synthesizes protein toxin as a result of colonization of vaginal tampons

**285.** An 18-year-old male patient presents to the emergency room with a 3-day history of fever, dry cough, difficulty breathing, and muscle aches and pains. His chest x-ray shows a diffuse left upper lobe infiltrate. *M. pneumoniae* pneumonia (walking pneumonia) may be rapidly identified by which of the following procedures?

a. Cold agglutinin test
b. Culture of respiratory secretions in HeLa cells after centrifugation of the inoculated tubes
c. Culture of respiratory secretions on monkey kidney cells
d. Detection of specific antigen in urine
e. Electron microscopy of sputum

**286.** Influenza can be treated; therefore, specific detection of the virus becomes much more important. Which of the following is best for detection of influenza?

a. Cold agglutinin test
b. Culture of respiratory secretions on monkey kidney cells
c. Detection of antigen in respiratory secretions
d. Detection of specific antigen in urine
e. Electron microscopy of sputum

**287.** A 50-year-old male presents with severe bilateral pulmonary infiltrate, elevated temperature leucocytosis, elevated enzymes, and elevated creatine kinase. He recently visited his favorite resturant that had a large water fountain that was misty on the day of his visit. Which of the following procedures would most rapidly diagnose the suspected organism that is the etiologic agent of Legionnaires' disease in this patient?

a. Cold agglutinin test
b. Culture of respiratory secretions on a charcoal-based nutrient agar
c. Detection of antigen in respiratory secretions
d. Detection of specific antigen in urine
e. Electron microscopy of sputum

**288.** *Chlamydia pneumoniae* has recently been implicated in respiratory disease primarily in children. Which of the following best isolates this fastidious bacterium?

a. Cold agglutinin test
b. Culture of respiratory secretions in HeLa cells after centrifugation of the inoculated tubes
c. Culture of respiratory secretions on monkey kidney cells
d. Detection of specific antigen in urine
e. Electron microscopy of sputum

**289.** A 5-year-old boy is brought to the local public health clinic because of a severe, intractable cough. During the previous 10 days, he had a persistent cold that had worsened. The cough developed the previous day and was so severe that vomiting frequently followed it. The child appears exhausted from the coughing episodes. A blood cell count shows a marked leukocytosis with a predominance of lymphocytes. Which of the following procedures can best detect the etiologic agent?

a. Cold agglutinin test
b. Culture of respiratory secretions in HeLa cells after centrifugation of the inoculated tubes
c. Culture of respiratory secretions on Bordet-Gengou agar
d. Direct microscopy of sputum by Gram stain
e. Fluorescent antibody detection of the organism in sputum

# Bacteriology

## *Answers*

**178. The answer is d.** (*Brooks, pp 275–276. Levinson, pp 141, 477s. Murray—2005, pp 353–354. Ryan, pp 381–383.*) *H. pylori* was first recognized as a possible cause of gastritis and peptic ulcer by Marshall and Warren in 1984. This organism is readily isolated from gastric biopsies but not from stomach contents. It is similar to *Campylobacter* species and grows on chocolate agar at 37°C in the same microaerophilic environment suitable for *C. jejuni* (Campy-Pak or anaerobic jar [Gas Pak] without the catalyst). *H. pylori*, however, grows more slowly than *C. jejuni*, requiring 5–7 days' incubation. *C. jejuni* grows optimally at 42°C, not 37°C, as does *H. pylori*.

| Diagnostic Tests for *Helicobacter pylori* | | |
|---|---|---|
| | **Advantages** | **Disadvantages** |
| **Noninvasive** | | |
| Serum ELISA | Inexpensive | Not useful for follow-up |
| Urea breath test | Useful for follow-up | Expensive; may be falsely negative in patients on acid suppression therapy |
| Stool antigen test | Inexpensive; useful for follow-up | Inconvenient |
| Whole blood assay | Inexpensive; rapid | Less accurate than serum ELISA* |
| **Invasive (endoscopic)** | | |
| Histology | Visualization of pathology | May miss low-grade infection |
| Rapid urease | Rapid | May be falsely positive in bacterial overgrowth |
| Culture | Antibiotic susceptibility | Not maximally sensitive; not available routinely; requires 4–7 d |

*Enzyme-linked immunosorbent assay.

*Reprinted, with permission, from Wilson WR, Sande MA.* Current Diagnosis and Treatment in Infectious Disease. *New York: McGraw-Hill, 2001: 584.*

**179. The answer is a.** (*Brooks, pp 279–281. Levinson, p 148. Murray—2005, pp 370–372. Ryan, pp 399–400.*) The major determinant of virulence in *H. influenzae* is the presence of a capsule. There is no demonstrable exotoxin, and the role of endotoxin is unclear. While one would expect that IgA protease would inhibit local immunity, the role of this enzyme in pathogenesis is as yet unclear. See the table below for a comparison of gram-neagtive rods associated with the respiratory tract.

**180. The answer is e.** (*Brooks, pp 248–252; 269. Levinson, pp 11, 41–44. Murray—2005, pp 323–339. Ryan, pp 348, 375.*) The toxin of *V. cholerae* and LT enterotoxin from *E. coli* are similar. The B subunits of the toxins bind to ganglioside GM1 receptors on the host cell. The A subunits catalyze transfer of the ADP-ribose moiety of ADP to a regulatory protein known as $G_s$. This activated $G_s$ stimulates adenyl cyclase. Cyclic AMP is increased, as is fluid and electrolyte release from the crypt cells into the lumen of the bowel. Watery, profuse diarrhea ensues.

**181. The answer is d.** (*Brooks, pp 316, 645–647. Levinson, pp 25, 182, 484s. Murray—2005, p 397. Ryan, p 904.*) Microscopic examination can readily demonstrate clue cells (epithelial cells with *Gardnerella* bacteria attached) or pseudohyphae (*Candida*). A wet mount will be needed to demonstrate motile *Trichomonas* cells. *Candida, Trichomonas,* and bacterial vaginitis are seen most often. *Staphylococcus aureus* is involved much less frequently. While *E. coli* may be a common cause of genitourinary infection, clue cells are usually absent. See the table below for a comparison of these bacteria.

**182. The answer is d.** (*Brooks, pp 223–230. Levinson, pp 104–105, 469s. Murray—2005, pp 221–236. Ryan, p 268.*) *S. aureus* is a well-known pathogen that is very opportunistic and commonly causes abscess lesions. It routinely may resist phagocytosis by WBCs due to protein A. Osteomyelitis and arthritis, either hematogenous or traumatic, are commonly caused by *S. aureus,* especially in children. *Salmonella* are gram-negative. *S. saprophyticus* is a common skin flora and is usually not pathogenic. *S. pneumoniae* is seldom or never involved in osteomyelitis infections, as is true for *L. monocytogenes.*

## GRAM-NEGATIVE RODS ASSOCIATED WITH THE RESPIRATORY TRACT

| Species | Major Diseases | Laboratory Diagnosis | Factors X and V Required for Growth | Vaccine Available | Prophylaxis for Contacts |
|---|---|---|---|---|---|
| H. influenzae | Meningitis*, otitis media, sinusitis, pneumonia, epiglottitis | Culture; capsular polysaccharide in serum or spinal fluid | + | + | Rifampin |
| B. pertussis | Whooping cough (pertussis) | Fluorescent antibody on secretions; culture | – | + | Erythromycin |
| L. pneumophila | Pneumonia | Serology; urinary antigen; culture | – | – | None |

*In countries where the H. influenzae b conjugate vaccine has been deployed, the vaccine has greatly reduced the incidence of meningitis caused by this organism.
Reprinted, with permission, from Levinson W, Jawetz E. Medical Microbiology and Immunology, 7e. New York: McGraw-Hill, 2002.

## CLINICAL FEATURES OF VAGINITIS

| | Normal | Vulvovaginal Candidiasis | Trichomoniasis | Bacterial Vaginosis |
|---|---|---|---|---|
| **Symptoms** | None | Pruritus<br>Soreness<br>Dyspareunia | Soreness<br>Dyspareunia<br>Often asymptomatic | Often asymptomatic<br>Occasional abdominal pain |
| **Discharge** | | | | |
| Amount | Variable | Scant/moderate | Profuse | Moderate |
| Color | Clear/white | White | Green-yellow | White/gray |
| Consistency | Nonhomogenous floccular | Clumped, adherent | Homogenous, frothy | Homogenous adherent |
| **Vaginal fluid pH** | 4.0–4.5 | 4.0–4.5 | 5.0–6.0 | >4.5 |
| **Amine test** (fish odor) | None | None | Usually positive | Positive |
| **Microscopy** | | | | |
| Saline | PMN:EC* ratio <1<br>Lactobacilli predominate | PMN:EC <1<br>Pseudohyphae (~40%) | PMN:EC >1<br>Motile trichomonads<br>PMNs predominate | PMN:EC <1<br>Clue cells<br>Coccobacilli |
| 10% KOH | Negative | Pseudohyphae (~70%) | Negative | Negative |

*PMN-Polymorphonuclear leukocytes; EC-vaginal epithelial cells.

Reprinted, with permission, from Wilson WR, Sande MA. Current Diagnosis and Treatment in Infectious Disease. *New York: McGraw-Hill, 2001:209.*

**183. The answer is c.** (*Brooks, p 293. Levinson, pp 129, 155, 480s. Murray—2005, pp 374–375. Ryan, p 490.*) *Pasteurella* (gram-negative coccobacilli) are primarily animal pathogens, but they can cause a wide range of human diseases. They have a bipolar appearance on stained smears. *P. multocida* occurs worldwide in domestic and wild animals. It is the most common organism in human wounds inflicted by bites of cats and dogs. It is a common cause of hemorrhagic septicemia in a variety of animals. Wounds commonly present with an acute onset (within hours) of redness, swelling, and pain. The other organisms are routinely found in the environment and may be opportunistic pathogens. *P. multocida* is a gram-negative rod that usually responds to penicillin treatment.

**184–186. The answers are 184-c, 185-a, 186-a.** (*Brooks, pp 343–347. Levinson, pp 166–167, 65. Murray—2005, pp 443–446. Ryan, pp 410–411.*) *M. pneumoniae* causes a respiratory infection known as primary atypical pneumonia, or walking pneumonia. Although disease caused by *M. pneumoniae* can be contracted year-round, thousands of cases occur during the winter months in all age groups. The disease, if untreated, will persist for 2 weeks or longer. Rare but serious side effects include cardiomyopathies and CNS complications. Infection with *M. pneumoniae* may be treated with either erythromycin or tetracycline. The organism lacks a cell wall and so is resistant to the penicillin and the cephalosporin groups of antibiotics.

Until recently, diagnostic tests have been of limited value. Up to 50% of cases may not show cold agglutinins, an insensitive and nonspecific acute-phase reactant. However, if cold agglutinins are present, a quick diagnosis can be made if signs and symptoms are characteristic. Complement fixation tests that measure an antibody to a glycolipid antigen of *M. pneumoniae* are useful but not routinely performed in most laboratories. Also, cross-reactions may occur. Culture of *M. pneumoniae*, while not technically difficult, may take up to 2 weeks before visible growth is observed.

A DNA probe is available. It is a 125I probe for the 16S ribosomal RNA of *M. pneumoniae*. Evaluations in a number of laboratories indicate that compared with culture it is highly sensitive and specific. Recently, DNA probes have been applied to the detection of *M. pneumoniae* in clinical specimens.

**187. The answer is a.** (*Brooks, pp 754–757. Levinson, pp 156–160. Murray—2005, pp 301–302. Ryan, pp 445–446.*) Most cases of tuberculosis are caused when patients inhale droplet nuclei containing infectious organisms. While the bacilli are deposited on the alveolar spaces, they do not clog up the alveoli but are engulfed by macrophages. Tissue injury is not a result of toxin secretion but of cell-mediated hypersensitivity, that is, "immunologic injury."

**188. The answer is c.** (*Brooks, pp 189–191. Levinson, pp 75–76. Murray—2005, pp 210–211. Ryan, p 33.*) A new class of antibiotics, the quinolones, has one member, nalidixic acid, that has been available for years. The new representatives are much more active biologically and are effective against virtually all gram-negative bacteria and most gram-positive bacteria. They include norfloxacin, ofloxacin, ciprofloxacin, enoxacin, and the fluorinated quinolones such as lomefloxacin. These antibiotics kill bacteria by inhibition of synthesis of nucleic acid, more specifically, DNA gyrase. Resistance to quinolones has been observed and appears to be a class-specific phenomenon. An exception is when an organism is resistant to nalidixic acid, elevated minimal inhibitory concentrations (MICs) will generally apply to other quinolones, although these MICs will still be within the range of susceptibility.

**189. The answer is c.** (*Brooks, pp 166, 225. Levinson, pp 103, 106, 112. Murray—2005, pp 44–45. Ryan, pp 269–270.*) VISA was first recognized in Japan. Emergence in the United States soon followed. It is likely that the human VISA isolates have resulted from increased use of vancomycin for patients with MRSA or perhaps an increased pool of VISA in the environment selected out by the use of glycopeptides such as avoparcin, a growth promoter used in food-producing animals. In patients with VISA, the Centers for Disease Control (CDC) strongly recommends compliance with isolation procedures and other infection control practices geared to control of VISA.

**190. The answer is a.** (*Brooks, pp 720, 739–740. Levinson, pp 61–62, 66. Murray—2005, p 843. Ryan, pp 854–855.*) Many sputum specimens are cultured unnecessarily. Sputum is often contaminated with saliva or is almost totally made up of saliva. These specimens rarely reveal the cause of the patient's respiratory problem and may provide laboratory information that is harmful. The sputum in the question appears to be a good specimen because there are few epithelial cells. The pleomorphic, gram-negative rods are suggestive of *Haemophilus,* but culture of the secretions is necessary. Normal flora from a healthy oral cavity consists of gram-positive cocci and rods, with few or no PMNs.

**191. The answer is b.** *(Brooks, pp 305–306. Levinson, pp 145–146, 478s. Murray—2005, pp 422–425. Ryan, pp 324–325.) B. fragilis* is a constituent of normal intestinal flora and readily causes wound infections often mixed with aerobic isolates. These anaerobic, gram-negative rods are uniformly resistant to aminoglycosides and usually to penicillin as well. Reliable laboratory identification may require multiple analytical techniques. Generally, wound exudates smell bad owing to production of organic acids by such anaerobes as *B. fragilis.* Black exudates or a black pigment (heme) in the isolated colony is usually a characteristic of *Bacteroides (Porphyromonas) melaninogenicus,* not *B. fragilis.* Potent neurotoxins are synthesized by the gram-positive anaerobes such as *C. tetani* and *C. botulinum.*

**192. The answer is b.** *(Brooks, pp 295–303. Levinson, pp 117–118. Murray— 2005, pp 315–318. Ryan, p 336.)* Typical *Neisseria* are gram-negative diplococci. *N. gonorrhoeae* contain pili, hairlike appendages that may be several micrometers long (see figure below). They enhance attachment of the organism to mucous membranes, helping to make the organism more resistant to phagocytosis by WBCs. Gonococci isolated from clinical specimens produce small colonies containing piliated bacteria. Capsules appear to be less important in gonococcal infection than *N. meningitidis* infections. Flagella, peptidoglycan, LPS, and F pili do not significantly relate to pathogenesis, other than that LPS (endotoxin) release may become significant later in infection.

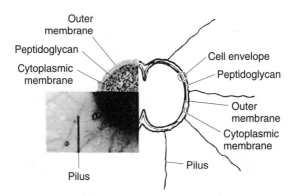

Collage and drawing of *N. gonorrhoeae* showing pili and the three layers of the cell envelope. *(Reproduced, with permission, from Brooks GF et al. Jawetz's Medical Microbiology, 23e. New York: McGraw-Hill, 2004:296.)*

**193. The answer is d.** (*Brooks, pp 217–218. Levinson, p 114. Murray—2005, pp 273–276. Ryan, pp 302–304.*) *Listeria* multiply both extracellularly and intracellularly, but under most circumstances a competent immune system eliminates *Listeria*. As expected, listeriosis is seen in the very young and the very old, and in people with compromised immune systems. Reports of *Listeria* food outbreaks have implicated such foods as coleslaw and milk products, especially if not pasteurized.

**194–197. The answers are 194–d, 195-a, 196-c, 197-d.** (*Brooks, pp 331–334. Levinson, pp 168–170. Murray—2005, pp 427–433. Ryan, pp 424–430.*) This patient appears to have primary syphilis, as evidenced by a penile chancre that was not tender. One of the differences between syphilis and herpes simplex virus (HSV) is that an HSV lesion is excruciatingly painful. Treponemal organisms may be seen microscopically in the lesion if the lesion is scraped. If not treated, the chancre will disappear and the patient will be asymptomatic until he/she exhibits the signs and symptoms of secondary syphilis, which include a disseminated rash and systemic involvement such as meningitis, hepatitis, or nephritis. There are two kinds of tests for the detection of syphilis antibodies: nonspecific tests such as the RPR and VDRL, and specific tests such as the FTA, *T. pallidum* hemagglutination test (TPHA), and the microhemagglutination—*T. pallidum* (MHTP). The difference is that the nonspecific tests use a cross-reactive antigen known as cardiolipin, while the specific tests use a *T. pallidum* antigen. Although the nonspecific tests are sensitive, they lack specificity and often cross-react in patients who have diabetes, hepatitis, or infectious mononucleosis, or who are pregnant. Some patients, especially those with autoimmune diseases, will have both nonspecific (RPR) and specific tests (FTA) positive even if they do not have syphilis. Resolution of such a situation can be done by molecular methods for *T. pallidum*, such as PCR, or by the immobilization test using live spirochetes and the patient's serum. In the TPI test, the spirochetes will die in the presence of specific antibody. (See figure below.)

**198. The answer is c.** (*Brooks, pp 312–314. Levinson, pp 32, 150–151. Murray—2005, pp 392–394. Ryan, pp 415–419.*) The symptoms of Legionnaires' disease are similar to those of mycoplasmal pneumonia and influenza. Affected persons are moderately febrile, complain of pleuritic chest pain, and have a dry cough. Unlike *Klebsiella* and *Staphylococcus*, *L. pneumophila* exhibits fastidious growth requirements. Charcoal yeast extract agar either with or without antibiotics is the preferred isolation medium.

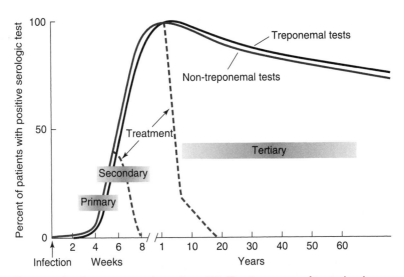

Treponemal and nontreponemal tests in syphilis. The time course of treated and untreated syphilis in relation to serologic tests is shown. The nontreponemal tests (VDRL, RPR) rise during primary syphilis and reach their peak in secondary syphilis. They slowly decline with advancing age. With treatment they revert to normal over a few weeks. The treponemal tests (FTA-Abs, MHTP) follow the same course but remain elevated even following successful treatment. (*Reprinted, with permission, from Ryan KJ et al. Sherris Medical Microbiology, 4e. New York: McGraw-Hill, 2001: 429.*)

While sputum may not be the specimen of choice for *Legionella*, the discovery of small, gram-negative rods by direct fluorescent antibody (FA) technique should certainly heighten suspicion of the disease. *L. pneumophila* is a facultative intracellular pathogen and enters macrophages without activating their oxidizing capabilities. The organisms bind to macrophage C receptors, which promote engulfment.

**199. The answer is b.** (*Brooks, pp 209–210. Levinson, pp 124, 473s–474s. Murray—2005, pp 411–413. Ryan, pp 322–324.*) Patients treated with antibiotics develop diarrhea that, in most cases, is self-limiting. However, in some instances, particularly in those patients treated with ampicillin or clindamycin, a severe, life-threatening pseudomembranous enterocolitis develops. This disease has characteristic histopathology, and membranous plaques can be seen in the colon by endoscopy. Pseudomembranous enterocolitis and antibiotic-associated diarrhea are caused by an anaerobic gram-positive rod,

*C. difficile.* It has been recently shown that *C. difficile* produces a protein toxin with a molecular weight of about 250,000. The "toxin" is, in fact, two toxins, toxin A and toxin B. Both toxins are always present in fecal samples, but there is approximately 1000 times more toxin B than toxin A. Toxin A has entero-toxic activity—that is, it elicits a positive fluid response in ligated rabbit ileal loops—whereas toxin B appears to be primarily a cytotoxin.

**200. The answer is b.** (*Brooks, pp 231–238, 217–218. Levinson, pp 126–127, 107–108. Murray—2005, pp 248–249, 273–276. Ryan, pp 286–287, 302–305.*) Group B streptococci are normal flora in a sizeable number of women, who show no vaginal adverse disease. *L. monocytogenes* also may be present as normal vaginal flora. Streptococci from clinical specimens usually grow in small, pinpoint colonies. *Listeria*, usually growing intracel-lularly in vivo, also produce small colonies on blood agar. Both also pro-duce β (clear zone) hemolysis. Of the proposed tests, catalase is easy to perform and interpret. Group B streptococci do not produce catalase, while *Listeria* are catalase-positive. See the table below for a comparison of medically-important streptococci.

| STREPTOCOCCI OF MEDICAL IMPORTANCE | | | |
|---|---|---|---|
| **Species** | **Lancefield Group** | **Typical Hemolysis** | **Diagnostic Features[1]** |
| *S. pyogenes* | A | β | Bacitracin-sensitive |
| *S. agalactiae* | B | β | Bacitracin-resistant; hippurate hydrolyzed |
| *E. faecalis* | D | α or β or none | Growth in 6.5% NaCl[3] |
| *S. bovis*[2] | D | α or none | No growth in 6.5% NaCl |
| *S. pneumoniae* | NA[4] | α | Bile-soluble; inhibited by optochin |
| Viridans group[5] | NA | α | Not bile-soluble; not inhibited by optochin |

[1]All streptococci are catalase-negative.
[2]*S. bovis* is a nonenterococcal group D organism.
[3]Both *E. faecalis* and *S. bovis* grow on bile-esculin agar, whereas other streptococci do not. They hydrolyze the esculin, and this results in a characteristic black discoloration of the agar.
[4]NA, not applicable.
[5]Viridans group streptococci include several species, such as *S. anguis, S. mutans, S. mitis, S. gordoni, S. sali-varius, S. anginosus, S. milleri,* and *S. intermedius.*

*Reprinted, with permission, from Levinson W, Jawetz E. Medical Microbiology and Immunology, 7e. New York: McGraw-Hill, 2002: 95.*

**201. The answer is a.** *(Brooks, pp 279–281. Levinson, p. 148. Murray— 2005, pp 370–374. Ryan, pp 397–401.)* Meningitis caused by *H. influenzae* cannot be distinguished on clinical grounds from that caused by pneumococci or meningococci. The symptoms described are typical for all three organisms. *H. influenzae* is a small, gram-negative rod with a polysaccharide capsule. It is able to grow on laboratory media if two factors are added. Heme (factor X) and NAD (factor V) provide for energy production. Use of the conjugate vaccine (type b polysaccharide) reduces the disease incidence more than 90%. Pneumococci are gram-positive diplococci, and meningococci are gram-negative diplococci, which grow on blood agar and chocolate agar with no X and V factors needed, respectively.

**202. The answer is a.** *(Brooks, pp 218–220. Levinson, pp 164–165, 481s–482s. Murray—2005, pp 417–419. Ryan, pp 458–459.)* The patient presented with typical symptoms of actinomycosis. *Actinomyces israelii* is normal flora in the mouth. However, it causes a chronic draining infection, often around the maxilla or the mandible, with osteomyelitic changes. Treatment is high-dose penicillin for 4–6 weeks. The diagnosis of actinomycosis is often complicated by the failure of *A. israelii* to grow from the clinical specimen. It is an obligate anaerobe. Fluorescent antibody (FA) reagents are available for direct staining of *A. israelii*. A rapid diagnosis can be made from the pus. FA conjugates are also available for *Actinomyces viscosis* and *A. odontolyticus*, anaerobic actinomycetes that are rarely involved in actinomycotic abscesses.

**203–205. The answers are 203-a, 204-b, 205-b.** *(Brooks, pp 231–238. Levinson, pp 107–109, 470s, 107–112. Murray—2005, pp 248–249. Ryan, pp 286–287.)* The incidence of GBS disease is 1–3 cases per 1000 births. Neonates acquire the disease during birth from mothers who harbor the organism. Risk factors include prematurity, premature rupture of membranes, and group B streptococcal carriage. The Gram stain of CSF is a rapid test for GBS disease. Although sensitive, the Gram stain requires experience to differentiate these streptococci from other gram-positive cocci. Latex tests for GBS antigen are also available, but sensitivity in CSF is not significantly higher than the Gram stain. GBS can be reduced by intrapartum administration of penicillin. While GBS is relatively more resistant to penicillin than group A streptococci, the great majority of GBS isolates are still penicillin-susceptible. An aminoglycoside such as gentamicin may be added to GBS treatment regimens due to the relative reduced susceptibility of some strains. Experimentally, GBS polysaccharide vaccines have also been used. Screening pregnant females early in pregnancy probably offers little advantage because of the possible acquisition of GBS late in the pregnancy. There has been speculation concerning the pathogenesis of GBS. This includes failure to activate complement pathways and immobilization of polymorphonuclear leukocytes due to the inactivation of complement C5a, a potent chemoattractant.

**206. The answer is a.** (*Brooks, pp 331–334. Levinson, pp 168–170. Murray— 2005, pp 427–433. Ryan, pp 424–429.*) In men, the appearance of a hard chancre on the penis characteristically indicates syphilis. Even though the chancre does not appear until the infection is 2 or more weeks old, the VDRL test for syphilis still can be negative despite the presence of a chancre (the VDRL test may not become positive for 2 or 3 weeks after initial infection). However, a lesion suspected of being a primary syphilitic ulcer should be examined by dark-field microscopy, which can reveal motile treponemes.

**207. The answer is a.** (*Brooks, pp 284–286. Levinson, pp 152, 479s–480s. Murray—2005, pp 383–385. Ryan, pp 483–484.*) *Brucella* are small, aerobic, gram-negative coccobacilli. Of the four well-characterized species of *Brucella*, only one—*B. melitensis*—characteristically infects both goats and humans. Brucellosis may be associated with gastrointestinal and neurologic symptoms, lymphadenopathy, splenomegaly, hepatitis, and osteomyelitis. Susceptibility to dyes (thionin and basic fuschin) can help in differentiation of the species. See the table below for a listing of gram-negative rods associated with animal sources.

| GRAM-NEGATIVE RODS ASSOCIATED WITH ANIMAL SOURCES | | | | |
|---|---|---|---|---|
| Species | Disease | Source of Human Infection | Mode of Transmission from Animal to Human | Diagnosis |
| *Brucella species* | Brucellosis | Pigs, cattle, goats, sheep | Dairy products; contact with animal tissues | Serology or culture |
| *F. tularensis* | Tularemia | Rabbits, deer, ticks | Contact with animal tissues; ticks | Serology |
| *Y. pestis* | Plague | Rodents | Flea bite | Immunofluorescence or culture |
| *P. multocida* | Cellulitis | Cats, dogs | Cat or dog bite | Wound culture |

*Reprinted, with permission, from Levinson W, Jawetz E.* Medical Microbiology and Immunology, *7e. New York: McGraw-Hill, 2002: 139.*

## SPIROCHETES OF MEDICAL IMPORTANCE

| Species | Disease | Mode of Transmission | Diagnosis | Morphology | Growth in Bacteriologic Media | Treatment |
|---|---|---|---|---|---|---|
| *T. pallidum* | Syphilis | Intimate (sexual) contact; across the placenta | Microscopy; serologic tests | Thin, tight, spirals, seen by dark-field illumination, silver impregnation, or immunofluorescent stain | — | Penicillin G |
| *B. burgdorferi* | Lyme disease | Tick bite | Clinical observations; microscopy | Large, loosely coiled; stain with Giemsa stain | + | Tetracycline or amoxicillin for acute; penicillin G for chronic |
| *B. recurrentis* | Relapsing fever | Louse bite | Clinical observations; microscopy | Large, loosely coiled; stain with Giemsa stain | + | Tetracycline |
| *L. interrogans* | Leptospirosis | Food or drink contaminated by urine of infected animals (rats, dogs, pigs, cows) | Serologic tests | Thin, tight spirals, seen by dark-field illumination | + | Penicillin G |

Reprinted, with permission, from Levinson W, Jawetz E. Medical Microbiology and Immunology. 7e. New York: McGraw-Hill, 2002:154.

**208. The answer is a.** (*Brooks, pp 270–272. Levinson, pp 19, 40–41, 139. Murray—2005, pp 340–341. Ryan, pp 376–377.*) Cholera is a toxicosis. The mode of action of cholera toxin is to stimulate the activity of adenyl cyclase, an enzyme that converts ATP to cyclic AMP. Cyclic AMP stimulates the secretion of chloride ion, and affected patients lose copious amounts of fluid. A drug that inhibits adenyl cyclase thus might block the effect of cholera toxin. Water and electrolyte replacement are primary management mechanisms, while oral tetracycline may help reduce stool output.

**209. The answer is d.** (*Brooks, pp 155, 225. Levinson, pp 44, 104. Murray— 2005, pp 228–233. Ryan, pp 263–264.*) Certain strains of staphylococci elaborate an enterotoxin that is frequently responsible for food poisoning. Typically, the toxin is produced when staphylococci grow on foods rich in carbohydrates and is present in the food when it is consumed. The resulting gastroenteritis is dependent only on the ingestion of toxin and not on bacterial multiplication in the gastrointestinal tract. Characteristic symptoms are nausea, vomiting, abdominal cramps, and explosive diarrhea. The illness rarely lasts more than 24 hours.

**210. The answer is e.** (*Brooks, pp 223–224. Levinson, pp 104–105. Murray— 2005, pp 44–45. Ryan, pp 269–270.*) Staphylococci are gram-positive, non-spore-forming cocci. Clinically, their antibiotic resistance poses major problems. Many strains produce β-lactamase (penicillinase), an enzyme that destroys penicillin by opening the lactam ring. Drug resistance, mediated by plasmids, may be transferred by transduction.

**211. The answer is c.** (*Brooks, pp 205–207. Levinson, pp 122–123, 473s. Murray—2005, pp 409–410. Ryan, pp 320–322.*) C. botulinum growing in food produces a potent neurotoxin that causes diplopia, dysphagia, respiratory paralysis, and speech difficulties when ingested by humans. The toxin is thought to act by blocking the action of acetylcholine at neuromuscular junctions. Botulism is associated with high mortality; fortunately, C. botulinum infection in humans is rare.

**212. The answer is a.** (*Brooks, pp 295–304. Levinson, pp 115–118. Murray— 2005, pp 315–319. Ryan, p 327.*) Several Neisseria species make up part of the normal (nonpathogenic) flora of the human upper respiratory tract. While commensal organisms seldom cause disease, they may occasionally be opportunistic. These organisms are also "foreign" to the immune system and cause immune responses to occur, especially humoral (antibody). The pathogens (*N. gonorrhae* and *N. meningitidis*) produce factors that ensure successful colonization of tissue in spite of local immune defense mechanisms.

**213. The answer is d.** *(Brooks, pp 273–275. Levinson, pp 140–141. Murray—2005, pp 347–351. Ryan, pp 379–380.)* Until recently, both erythromycin and ciprofloxacin were the drugs of choice for *C. jejuni* enterocolitis. Recently, resistance to the quinolones (ciprofloxacin) has been observed. Ampicillin is ineffective against this gram-negative, curved rod. While Pepto-Bismol may be adequate for a related ulcer-causing bacterium, *Helicobacter,* it is not used for *C. jejuni.* While the pathogenesis of *C. jejuni* suggests an enterotoxin, an antitoxin is not available.

**214. The answer is b.** *(Brooks, pp 279–281. Levinson, p 148. Murray—2005, pp 370–373. Ryan, pp 397–401.)* **H.** *influenzae* is a gram-negative bacillus. In young children, it can cause pneumonitis, sinusitis, otitis, and meningitis. Occasionally, it produces a fulminative laryngotracheitis with such severe swelling of the epiglottis that tracheostomy becomes necessary. Clinical infections with this organism after the age of 3 years are less frequent, especially since approval of the type b vaccine.

**215–217. The answers are 215-a, 216-d, 217-e.** *(Brooks, pp 242–244. Levinson, pp 27, 470s–471s, 108. Murray—2005, pp 259–262. Ryan, pp 294–295.)* Enterococci cause a wide variety of infections ranging from less serious—for example, urinary tract infections—to very serious, such as septicemia. A gram-positive coccus resistant to penicillin must be assumed to be enterococcus until other, more definitive biochemical testing places the isolate in one of the more esoteric groups of gram-positive cocci. Once isolated, there are a variety of tests to speciate enterococci. However, penicillin-resistant, non-β-lactamase-producing, vancomycin-resistant, gram-positive cocci are most likely *E. faecium.* There are a variety of mechanisms for vancomycin resistance in *E. faecium,* and they have been termed Van A, B, or C. These isolates have become one of the most feared nosocomial pathogens in the hospital environment. Unfortunately, no approved antibiotics can successfully treat vancomycin-resistant enterococci (VRE)—only some experimental antibiotics such as Synercid.

**218. The answer is c.** *(Brooks, pp 750–751. Levinson, pp 105, 508. Murray—2005, pp 232–233. Ryan, p 824.)* S. aureus is implicated in the majority of cases of acute osteomyelitis, which affects children most often. A superficial staphylococcal lesion frequently precedes the development of bone infection. In the preantibiotic era, S. pneumoniae was a common cause of acute osteomyelitis. M. tuberculosis and gram-negative organisms are implicated less frequently in this infection.

**219. The answer is c.** *(Brooks, pp 212–216. Levinson, pp 125–126, 474s. Murray—2005, pp 280–282. Ryan, p 170.)* All toxigenic strains of *Corynebacterium diphtheriae* are lysogenic for β-phage carrying the *Tox* gene, which codes for the toxin molecule. The expression of this gene is controlled by the metabolism of the host bacteria. The greatest amount of toxin is produced by bacteria grown on media containing very low amounts of iron. Fragment B of the toxin is required for cell entry, while Fragment A stops protein production by inhibiting elongation factor 2 (EF-2).

**220–222. The answers are 220-e, 221-e, 222-b.** *(Brooks, pp 154, 226. Levinson, pp 40–44, 104. Murray—2005, pp 226, 230. Ryan, pp 264–266.)* TSS is a febrile illness seen predominantly, but not exclusively, in menstruating women. Clinical criteria for TSS include fever greater than 102°F (38.9°C), rash, hypotension, and abnormalities of the mucous membranes and the gastrointestinal, hepatic, muscular, cardiovascular, or CNS. Usually 3 or more systems are involved. Treatment is supportive, including the aggressive use of antistaphylococcal antibiotics. Certain types of tampons may play a role in TSS by trapping $O_2$ and depleting magnesium. Most people have protective antibodies to the toxic shock syndrome toxin (TSST-1).

TSS is caused by a toxin-producing strain of S. aureus (TSST-1). In this case no actual organisms would likely be isolated since TSS is caused by an excreted toxin, not the actual organism. Blood culture would also most likely be negative. While there have been reports that S. epidermidis produces TSS, they have largely been discounted. Vaginal colonization with S. aureus is a necessary adjunct to the disease. S. aureus is isolated from the vaginal secretions, conjunctiva, nose, throat, cervix, and feces in 45–98% of cases. The organism has infrequently been isolated from the blood.

Epidemiologic investigations suggest strongly that TSS is related to use of tampons, in particular, use of the highly absorbent ones that can be left in for extended periods of time. An increased growth of intravaginal *Staphylococcus aureus* and enhanced production of TSST-1 have been associated with the prolonged intravaginal use of these hyperabsorbent tampons and with the capacity of the materials used in them to bind magnesium. The most severe cases of TSS have been seen in association with gram-negative infection. TSST-1 may enhance endotoxin activity. Recently, group A streptococci have been reported to cause TSS.

**223–224. The answers are 223-c, 224-d.** Bayesian statistics are often used to determine sensitivity, specificity, and predictive values of new diagnostic tests. A square is set up and the experimental numbers inserted: a = true positive, b = false positive, c = false negative, and d = true negative. The formulas for sensitivity, specificity, and predictive values are also given. (See figure below.)

It is necessary to note that the incidence of the disease in the population affects predictive values but not sensitivity or specificity. At a given level of sensitivity and specificity, as the incidence of the disease in the population increases, the predictive value of a positive (PVP) increases, and the predictive value of a negative (PVN) decreases. For this reason, predictive values are difficult to interpret unless true disease incidence is known.

|  | **Culture** | |
| --- | --- | --- |
| **LA Test** | **Pos** | **Neg** |
| POS | (a) 25 | (b) 5 |
| NEG | (c) 5 | (d) 95 |

$$\text{Sensitivity} = \frac{a}{a+c} = \frac{25}{25+5} = 85\%$$

$$\text{Specificity} = \frac{d}{d+b} = \frac{95}{95+5} = 95\%$$

$$\text{PVP} = \frac{a}{a+b} = \frac{25}{25+5} = 85\%$$

$$\text{PVN} = \frac{d}{d+c} = \frac{95}{95+5} = 95\%$$

**225. The answer is d.** (*Brooks, pp 262–264. Levinson, pp 142–145. Murray—2005, pp 357–366. Ryan, pp 387–388.*) Pseudomonads occur widely in soil, water, plants, and animals. They are gram-negative, motile, aerobic rods that produce water-soluble pigments (blue and green). They are very opportunistic when abnormal host defenses are encountered. While motile, they do not "swarm" over the surface of an agar plate, as *Proteus* does. Being gram-negative, as many enteric and environmental organisms are, their cell walls contain endotoxin (LPS). Many of the pseudomonads are resistant to a wide range of antimicrobials, enhancing their opportunistic characteristics.

**226. The answer is c.** (*Brooks, pp 202–211. Levinson, pp 119–124. Murray—2005, pp 265–272, 401–410. Ryan, pp 308, 314–317.*) *Clostridium* and *Bacillus* organisms exist widely in nature. While many *Clostridium* are pathogenic due to exotoxin production (*Clostridium tetanis, C. botulism*), and anthrax has multiple virulence factors (capsule, LF, EF, and PA), *C. perfringens* and *B. cereus* are found routinely in gastroenteritis outbreaks. Since both are sporeformers, the usual epidemiological investigation finds that heating foods kills vegetative bacteria but not spores. If food is inappropriately stored (>40°F–140°F), spores may germinate into vegetative bacteria and be ingested, causing the disease. Most episodes are self-limited. Both produce enterotoxins that account for similar disease presentations.

**227. The answer is e.** (*Brooks, pp 166, 228. Levinson, pp 74, 103, 106. Murray—2005, pp 44–45. Ryan, pp 269–270.*) The incidence of oxacillin- and MRSA has been rapidly increasing. MRSA and methicillin-sensitive *S. aureus* (MSSA) coexist in heterologous populations. Treatment of a patient harboring this heterologous population may provide a selective environment for the MRSA. Prior to changing therapy, the susceptibility of the isolate should be determined. Vancomycin has often been used effectively for MRSA, but it is expensive and nephrotoxic. There is no evidence that MRSA is any more virulent or invasive than susceptible strains. See the table below for a listing of medically-important staphylcocci.

| STAPHYLOCOCCI OF MEDICAL IMPORTANCE | | | | |
|---|---|---|---|---|
| **Species** | **Coagulase Production** | **Typical Hemolysis** | **Important Features\*** | **Typical Disease** |
| *S. aureus* | + | Beta | Protein A on surface | Abscess, food poisoning, toxic shock syndrome |
| *S. epidermidis* | – | None | Sensitive to novobiocin | Infection of prosthetic heart valves and hips; common member of skin flora |
| *S. saprophyticus* | – | None | Resistant to novobiocin | Urinary tract infection |

\*All staphylococci are catalase-positive.

*Reprinted, with permission, from Levinson W, Jawetz E.* Medical Microbiology and Immunology, *7e. New York: McGraw-Hill, 2002: 92.*

**228. The answer is b.** *(Levinson, pp 359–360. Murray—2005, pp 856–858.)* Coccidian-like bodies have been identified in stools of some patients with diarrhea. These organisms appear to be similar to blue-green algae and were referred to as *Cyanobacterium*-like until they were recently reclassified as *Cyclospora*. They are larger than the microsporidia and resemble neither *Giardia* nor *Prototheca* nor other algae-like organisms. Unlike *Cryptosporidium*, these organisms fluoresce under ultraviolet light. The diarrhea can be prolonged and relapsing, and the treatment is usually trimethoprim-sulfamethoxazole. See the figure below for an illustration of *Giardia lamblia*.

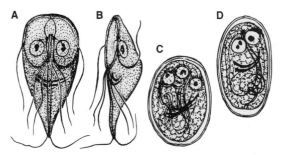

*Giardia lamblia.* A: "Face" and B: "profile" of vegetative forms; C and D: cysts (binucleate [D] and quadrinucleate stages). 2000 ×. *(Reproduced, with permission, from Brooks GF et al.* Jawetz's Medical Microbiology, *23e. New York: McGraw-Hill, 2001: 562.)*

**229. The answer is c.** (*Brooks, pp 252–253. Levinson, pp 131–134, 474s–475s. Murray—2005, pp 326–330. Ryan, pp 355–357.*) Food poisoning with *Escherichia coli* 0157/H7 causes hemorrhagic colitis; it is often seen in people who have eaten beef hamburgers. The same organism also causes a hemorrhagic uremic syndrome. The toxin, called *Shiga-like toxin*, can be demonstrated in Vero cells, but the cytotoxicity must be neutralized with specific antiserum. With the exception of sorbitol fermentation, there is nothing biochemically distinctive about these organisms.

**230. The answer is b.** (*Brooks, pp 252–253. Levinson, pp 131–134. Murray—2005, pp 326–330. Ryan, pp 355–357.*) ETEC is an important cause of traveler's diarrhea, producing a heat-labile exotoxin (LT) and a heat-stable enterotoxin (ST). To cause diarrhea, *E. coli* must produce not only LT and ST toxins but also adhere to the lining of the small intestine. Fimbrial antigens are involved in adherence. O657/H7 stain is called EHEC, while EPEC is also an important cause of diarrhea in infants. EIEC produces a shigellosis-type disease.

**231. The answer is d.** (*Brooks, pp 290–292. Levinson, pp 154–155. Murray—2005, pp 334–335. Ryan, pp 484–488.*) Bubonic plague and pneumonic plague differ clinically. Bubonic plague, characterized by swollen lymph nodes and fever, is usually transmitted through a flea bite. Pneumonic plague, which is characterized by sepsis and pneumonia, is transmitted by the droplet route, usually after contact with an infected human or animal.

**232. The answer is a.** (*Brooks, pp 214, 315. Levinson, pp 179–180, 484s. Murray—2005, p 398. Ryan, p 479.*) While the essential information (i.e., the evidence that the child in question was scratched by a cat) is missing, the clinical presentation points to a number of diseases, including cat-scratch disease (CSD). Until recently, the etiologic agent of CSD was unknown. Evidence indicated that it was a pleomorphic, rod-shaped bacterium that had been named *Afipia*. It was best demonstrated in the affected lymph node by a silver impregnation stain. However, it now appears that *Afipia* causes relatively few cases of CSD and that the free-living rickettsia primarily responsible is *Rochalimaea henselae*, which has recently been renamed *B. henselae*.

**233. The answer is c.** (*Brooks, pp 336–340. Levinson, pp 107–111. Murray—2005, pp 243–245. Ryan, p 273.*) There has been a marked increase in fatal streptococcal infections, including those that are described as "necrotizing fasciitis." The strains of group A streptococci isolated have a pyrogenic exotoxin with properties not unlike those of the toxic shock toxin of *S. aureus*. Mortality is high (30%) in spite of aggressive antibiotic therapy.

**234. The answer is b.** (*Brooks, pp 275–276. Levinson, pp 141, 477s. Murray— 2005, pp 353–354. Ryan, pp 383–384.*) *H. pylori* antigen tests from a stool sample using an ELISA format and a monoclonal antibody to *H. pylori* are as sensitive as culture of the control portion of the stomach. Urea breath tests are also widely used. *H. pylori* has an active enzyme (urease) that breaks down radioactive urea. The patient releases radioactive $CO_2$ if *H. pylori* are present. *H. pylori* antibody tests, IgG and IgA, indicate the presence of *H. pylori* and usually decline after effective treatment. Culture of stomach contents is insensitive and not appropriate as a diagnostic procedure for *H. pylori*. Direct tests such as antigen or culture of gastric mucosa are preferred because they are the most sensitive indication of a cure.

**235. The answer is e.** (*Brooks, pp 336–338. Levinson, pp 24, 170–172. Murray—2005, pp 433–436. Ryan, pp 434–437.*) At the present time, Lyme disease may be diagnosed clinically and serologically. Patients who are from endemic areas such as eastern Pennsylvania and report joint pain and swelling months subsequent to exposure to ticks must be evaluated for Lyme disease and treated if the test is positive. Patients may also report a variety of neurologic problems such as tingling of the extremities, Bell's palsy, and headache. IgM antibody appears soon after the tick bite (10 days to 3 weeks) and persists for 2 months; IgG appears later in the disease but remains elevated for 1–2 years, especially in untreated patients. A significant IgG titer is at least 1:320. Most investigators feel that IgM titers of 1:100 are significant; some investigators say that any IgM titer is significant. Management of this patient would best be done by immediately starting treatment with tetracycline, effective against *Borrelia burgdorferi*.

**236. The answer is c.** (*Brooks, pp 326–327. Levinson, pp 156–163. Murray— 2005, pp 303–305. Ryan, p 613.*) There are some interesting characteristics of *M. avium* from AIDS patients. According to data from the National Jewish Hospital and Research Center in Denver and the CDC, 75% of the isolates were serovar 4, and 76% produced a deep-yellow pigment. Yellow pigment is not a characteristic of most isolates of *M. avium*. The significance of these findings is unknown. Most *M. avium* isolates are resistant to isoniazid and streptomycin but susceptible to clofazimine and ansamycin. In vitro susceptibility testing, however, may not be reliable for *M. avium*. A blood culture is often the most reliable way to diagnose the disease.

**237. The answer is b.** *(Brooks, p 238. Levinson, pp 48, 111, 455. Murray— 2005, pp 244–245. Ryan, p 279.)* Rheumatic fever (RF) is a disease that causes polyarthritis, carditis, chorea, and erythema marginatum. The mechanism of damage appears to be autoimmune; that is, antibodies are synthesized to a closely related streptococcal antigen such as M-protein, but these same antibodies cross-react with certain cardiac antigens such as myosin. Until recently, RF was very rare in the United States. In 1986, there were at least 135 cases of RF in Utah. Subsequently, scattered cases of RF have occurred in other states. Epidemiologists do not have a reason for this increase in RF. Some evidence suggests that there may be a genetic predisposition to the disease. Intramuscular injection of benzathine penicillin is effective treatment for and prophylaxis against group A streptococcal infection.

**238. The answer is d.** *(Brooks, pp 233–236. Levinson, pp 108–109. Murray— 2005, pp 251–252. Ryan, pp 293–294.)* In the healthy oral cavity, gram-positive, α-hemolytic streptococci make up the predominant flora. Any dental manipulation causes bleeding, allowing the oral flora to get into the blood (bacteremia). Phagocytic activity by WBCs usually clears this in a few minutes. However, these same organisms are quite efficient at attaching to and colonizing heart valve defects. *S. viridians* is a typical member of this α-hemolytic group and is commonly found in subacute bacterial endocarditis.

**239. The answer is c.** *(Brooks, p 688. Levinson, pp 365–366. Murray— 2005, pp 912–913. Ryan, pp 799–801.)* *Echinococcus* is a small, three-segmented tapeworm found only in the intestines of dogs and other carnivores. Eggs leave these hosts and infect grazing animals. In the herbivore gut, the eggs hatch and the released forms penetrate the gut. Various organs (especially the liver) develop huge, fluid-filled cysts in which future scoleces form (hydatid sand). Dogs become infected when they feed on viscera of diseased sheep or cows. Hydatid disease in humans occurs only through ingestion of dog feces. Humans are only an intermediate host of this organism and never the final host. None of the other options are cestodes, or tapeworms.

**240. The answer is e.** *(Brooks, pp 241–242. Levinson, pp 112–114, 471. Murray—2005, p 256. Ryan, p 291.)* The quellung test determines the presence of bacterial capsules. Specific antibody is mixed with the bacterial suspension or with clinical material. The polysaccharide capsule-antibody complex is visible microscopically. The test is also termed *capsular swelling.* The capsules of *S. pneumoniae* as well as *N. meningitidis, H. influenzae,* and *K. pneumoniae* play a role in the pathogenicity of the organisms. These surface structures inhibit phagocytosis, perhaps by preventing attachment of the leukocyte pseudopod. *C. diphtheriae, Enterobacter,* and *H. parainfluenzae* are nonencapsulated.

**241. The answer is b.** *(Brooks, pp 279–281. Levinson, pp 24, 34, 76, 112–113, 147–148. Murray—2005, pp 369–371. Ryan, pp 302–305.)* No vaccine is available for *Listeria.* Except during a meningococcal epidemic, *H. influenzae* is the most common cause of bacterial meningitis in children. The organism is occasionally found to be associated with respiratory tract infections or otitis media. *H. influenzae, N. meningitidis, S. pneumoniae,* and *Listeria* account for 80–90% of all cases of bacterial meningitis. A purified polysaccharide vaccine conjugated to protein for *H. influenzae* type B is available. A tetravalent vaccine is available for *N. meningitidis* and a 23-serotype vaccine for *S. pneumoniae.*

**242–245. The answers are 242-e, 243-d, 244-a, 245-b.** *(Brooks, p 148. Levinson, pp 32–38. Murray—2005, p 193.)* Organisms may be transmitted in a number of ways, such as by air, food, hands, sexual contact, and infected needles. However, for each disease or disease category, there is usually a portal of entry not always unique to the organism. The skin is a tough integument and, infact, is resistant to most infectious organisms except those that may break down human skin. Breaches of the skin as by wounds, burns, and the like predispose patients to a variety of infections such as tetanus caused by wound contamination with spores of *C. tetani,* or direct infection by *Staphylococcus, Streptococcus,* or gram-negative rods (such as *Serratia* or *Pseudomonas*). The respiratory tract is a common portal of entry to such airborne organisms as *M. tuberculosis.* This is why respiratory precautions must be taken when patients are harboring viable *M. tuberculosis.* The gastrointestinal tract is usually infected from ingestion of contaminated food or water (*Shigella, Salmonella, Campylobacter*) or by an alteration of the normal microbial flora such as with *C. difficile* disease.

The genital tract may become infected either by sexual contact or by alteration of the genital environment, as often occurs with yeast infections. Several bacteria such as *N. gonorrhoeae*, *Chlamydia*, and *T. pallidum* are transmitted by direct sexual contact with infected partners.

**246–247. The answers are 246-d, 247-b.** (*Brooks, pp 266, 267. Levinson, pp 180–183. Murray—2005, pp 365, 399. Ryan, pp 390–391.*) While admittedly rare in human medicine, the bacteria referred to should be appreciated for their role in human disease. *Branhamella* is a gram-negative diplococcus. It has recently been renamed *Moraxella catarrhalis*. While it is a member of the normal flora, it may cause severe upper and lower respiratory tract infection, particularly in the immunosuppressed patient. Most isolates produce β-lactamase and are resistant to penicillin. *Capnocytophaga* grows best in a carbon dioxide atmosphere, as the name implies. It is isolated frequently from patients with periodontal disease but may also cause septicemia in susceptible patients. Rat-bite fever is caused by *Spirillum*, and the agent of (CSD) is *B. henselae*.

**248. The answer is b.** (*Brooks, pp 352–354. Levinson, pp 93, 177, 484s. Murray—2005, pp 459–461. Ryan, pp 477–478.*) *Coxiella burnetii* is a rickettsial organism that causes upper respiratory infections in humans. These can range from subclinical infection to influenza-like disease and pneumonia. Transmission to humans occurs from inhalation of dust contaminated with rickettsiae from placenta, dried feces, urine, or milk, or from aerosols in slaughterhouses. *C. burnetii* can also be found in ticks, which can transmit the agent to sheep, goats, and cattle. No skin rash occurs in these infections. Treatment includes tetracycline and chloramphenicol.

**249–251. The answers are 249-a, 250-d, 251-b.** (*Brooks, pp 242–244, 218–220. Levinson, pp 27, 83, 470s–471s. Murray—2005, pp 260–262, 417–418. Ryan, pp 294, 457–459, 870–871.*) These questions demonstrate commonly occurring clinical infectious diseases and microbiologic problems. Enterococci may be resistant to ampicillin and gentamicin. Vancomycin would be the drug of choice. However, laboratory results do not always correlate well with clinical response. The National Committee on Clinical Laboratory Standards recommends testing enterococci only for ampicillin and vancomycin. Some symptomatic patients may have 10 leukocytes per mL of urine but relatively few bacteria. The patient is likely infected and the organisms, particularly if in pure culture, should be further processed.

The patient in question 251 probably has actinomycosis. These laboratory data are not uncommon. There is no reason to work up all the contaminating bacteria. A fluorescent microscopy test for *A. israelii* is available. If positive, the FA provides a rapid diagnosis. In any event, it may be impossible to recover *A. israelii* from such a specimen. High-dose penicillin has been used to treat actinomycosis.

**252–256. The answers are 252-c, 253-d, 254-b, 255-d, 256-e.** *(Brooks, pp 170, 714–715. Levinson, pp 67–81. Murray—2005, pp 204–207. Ryan, p 195.)* There are few bacteria for which antimicrobial susceptibility is highly predictable. However, some agents are the drug of choice because of their relative effectiveness. Among the three antibiotics that have been shown to treat legionellosis effectively (erythromycin, rifampin, and minocycline), erythromycin is clearly superior, even though in vitro studies show the organism to be susceptible to other antibiotics.

Penicillin remains the drug of choice for *S. pneumoniae* and the group A streptococci, although a few isolates of penicillin-resistant pneumococci have been observed. Resistance among the pneumococci is either chromosomally mediated, in which case the minimal inhibitory concentrations (MICs) are relatively low, or plasmid-mediated, which results in highly resistant bacteria. The same is generally true for *H. influenzae*. Until the mid-1970s, virtually all isolates of *H. influenzae* were susceptible to ampicillin. There has been a rapidly increasing incidence of ampicillin-resistant isolates—almost 35–40% in some areas of the United States. Resistance is ordinarily mediated by β-lactamase, although ampicillin-resistant, β-lactamase-negative isolates have been seen. No resistance to penicillin has been seen in group A streptococci.

Lyme disease, caused by *B. burgdorferi*, has been treated with penicillin, erythromycin, and tetracycline. Treatment failures have been observed. Ceftriaxone has become the drug of choice, particularly in the advanced stages of Lyme disease.

*C. difficile* causes toxin-mediated pseudomembranous enterocolitis as well as antibiotic-associated diarrhea. Pseudomembranous enterocolitis is normally seen during or after administration of antibiotics. One of the few agents effective against *C. difficile* is vancomycin. Alternatively, bacitracin can be used.

**257–260. The answers are 257-a, 258-d, 259-b, 260-c.** (*Brooks, pp 269–278. Levinson, pp 128–146. Murray—2005, pp 339–356. Ryan, pp 373–378.*) Some organisms originally thought to be vibrios, such as *C. jejuni,* have been reclassified. *C. jejuni,* which grows best at 42°C, has its reservoir in birds and mammals and causes gastroenteritis in humans.

*V. cholerae* causes cholera, which is worldwide in distribution. The three serotypes for cholera are Ogawa (AB), Inaba (AC), and Hikojima (ABC). The isolate of *V. cholerae* is "string-test"-positive.

*V. parahaemolyticus* is a halophilic marine vibrio that causes gastroenteritis in humans, primarily from ingestion of cooked seafood. It is lactose-negative and sucrose-negative.

*V. vulnificus* is also halophilic. It has been suggested that these halophilic vibrios do not belong in the genus *Vibrio* but in the genus *Beneckea. V. vulnificus* is lactose-positive and produces heat-labile, extracellular toxin. Organisms that, unlike *V. cholerae,* do not agglutinate in 0-1 antiserum were once called nonagglutinable (NAG), or noncholera (NC), vibrios. Such a classification can be confusing because *V. vulnificus,* which is an NCV, nevertheless causes severe cholera-like disease. In addition, *V. vulnificus* can produce wound infections, septicemia, meningitis, pneumonia, and keratitis.

**261–264. The answers are 261-b, 262-d, 263-a, 264-e.** (*Brooks, pp 279–294. Levinson, pp 152–155. Murray—2005, pp 383–390. Ryan, pp 401–402, 481–488.*) The organisms described in the questions all are short, ovoid, gram-negative rods. For the most part, they are nutritionally fastidious and require blood or blood products for growth. These and related organisms are unique among bacteria in that, though they have an animal reservoir, they can be transmitted to humans. Humans become infected by a variety of routes, including ingestion of contaminated animal products (*B. abortus* in cattle), direct contact with contaminated animal material or with infected animals themselves (*Y. enterocolitica* and *B. bronchiseptica* in dogs), and animal bites (*P. multocida* in many different animals). The laboratory differentiation of these microbes may be difficult and must rely on a number of parameters, including biochemical and serologic reactions, development of specific antibody response in affected persons, and epidemiologic evidence of infection.

**265–267. The answers are 265-d, 266-e, 267-b.** (*Brooks, pp 62–70. Levinson, pp 60–66. Murray—2005, pp 25–34. Ryan, pp 339, 373, 449.*) The medium of choice for the isolation of pathogenic Neisseriae is Thayer-Martin (TM) agar. TM agar is both a selective and an enriched medium; it contains hemoglobin, the supplement Isovitalex, and the antibiotics vancomycin, colistin, nystatin, and trimethoprim. *V. cholerae* as well as other vibrios, including *V. parahaemolyticus* and *V. alginolyticus,* are isolated best on thiosulfate citrate bile salts sucrose medium, although media such as mannitol salt agar also support the growth of vibrios. Maximal growth occurs at a pH of 8.5–9.5 and at 37°C incubation. Löwenstein-Jensen slants or plates, which are composed of a nutrient base and egg yolk, are used routinely for the initial isolation of mycobacteria. Small inocula of *M. tuberculosis* can also be grown in oleic acid albumin media; large inocula can be cultured on simple synthetic media.

**268. The answer is b.** *(Brooks, pp 205–207. Levinson, pp 122–123. Murray—2005, pp 409–411. Ryan, pp 320–322.)* Botulism is a disease brought about by ingesting a preformed toxin. Anaerobic bacteria have grown in food, deposited the botulism toxin, and died. The toxin affects the CNS by inhibiting the release of acetylcholine at the neuronal synapse. This results in a flaccid paralysis and death by respiratory failure. At no stage of the disease will any antibiotic be able to modify or arrest the disease. Antitoxins (A, B, E) must be promptly administered, and ventilation assisted mechanically. In all other choices, antibiotics will provide a mechanism to kill or inhibit the microorganisms, bringing the infection under control.

**269. The answer is d.** *(Brooks, pp 338–340. Levinson, pp 99, 100, 172, 483s. Murray—2005, pp 438–441. Ryan, pp 430–431.)* Leptospirosis is a zoonosis of worldwide distribution. Human infection results from ingestion of water or food contaminated with leptospirae. Rats, mice, wild rodents, dogs, swine, and cattle excrete the organisms in urine and feces during active illness and during an asymptomatic carrier state. Drinking, swimming, bathing, or food consumption may lead to human infection. Children acquire the disease from dogs more often than do adults. Treatment can include doxycycline, ampicillin, or amoxicillin. Symptoms in humans range from fever and rash to jaundice through aseptic meningitis.

**270–273. The answers are 270-e, 271-a, 272-b, 273-d.** *(Brooks, pp 196–203. Levinson, pp 103–114, 145–146, 180–182. Murray—2005, pp 83–88. Ryan, p 143.)* An understanding of normal, or indigenous, microflora is essential in order to appreciate the abnormal. Usually, anatomic sites contiguous to mucous membranes are not sterile and have characteristic normal flora.

The skin flora differs as a function of location. Skin adjacent to mucous membranes may share some of the normal flora of the gastrointestinal system. Overall, the predominant bacteria on the skin surface are *S. epidermidis* and *Propionibacterium,* an anaerobic diphtheroid.

The mouth is part of the gastrointestinal tract, but its indigenous flora shows some distinct differences. While anaerobes are present in large numbers, particularly in the gingival crevice, the eruption of teeth at 6–9 months of age leads to colonization by organisms such as *S. mutans* and *Streptococcus sanguis,* both α-hemolytic streptococci. An edentulous person loses β-hemolytic streptococci as normal flora.

The gastrointestinal tract is sterile at birth and soon develops characteristic flora as a function of diet. In the adult, anaerobes such as *B. fragilis* and *Bifidobacterium* may outnumber coliforms and enterococci by a ratio of 1000:1. The colon contains $10^{11}$–$10^{12}$ bacteria per gram of feces.

Soon after birth, the vagina becomes colonized by lactobacilli. As the female matures, lactobacilli may still be predominant, but anaerobic cocci, diphtheroids, and anaerobic, gram-negative rods also are found as part of the indigenous flora. Changes in the chemical or microbiologic ecology of the vagina can have marked effects on normal flora and may promote infection such as vaginitis or vaginosis.

**274–277. The answers are 274-c, 275-d, 276-a, 277-e.** (*Brooks, pp 196–203. Levinson, pp 103–113, 164, 149–150. Murray—2005, pp 83–88. Ryan, pp 274–275, 457–459.*) *S. salivarius, S. mutans, Actinomyces israelii,* and *Actinomyces viscosis* are all part of the normal microbiota of the human mouth. Both genera are common causes of bacterial endocarditis. *S. mutans* is highly cariogenic (i.e., capable of producing dental caries), in large part because of its unique ability to synthesize a dextran bioadhesive that sticks to teeth. *S. salivarius* settles onto the mucosal epithelial surfaces of the human mouth soon after birth and is often found in the saliva. Members of the genus *Actinomyces* that are clinically significant can be differentiated by specific fluorescent antibody microscopy as well as a battery of physiologic tests, such as those assessing requirements for oxygen. *Actinomyces* organisms are opportunistic members of the normal oral microbiota. Both *A. israelii* and *Actinomyces viscosis* are pathogenic and can cause osteomyelitis in the cervicofacial region. Of the two species, *A. israelii*, which is anaerobic, is the more common causative agent of actinomycosis. *Actinomyces viscosis*, a facultative anaerobe, appears to be cariogenic.

**278–284. The answers are 278-b, 279-a, 280-e, 281-d, 282-c, 283-c, 284-a.** (*Brooks, pp 212–216, 282–283, 252–253. Levinson, pp 125–126, 148–150, 153–154. Murray—2005, pp 279–283, 378–381, 326–330.*) Diphtheria, a disease caused by *C. diphtheriae*, usually begins as a pharyngitis associated with pseudomembrane formation and lymphadenopathy. Growing organisms lysogenic for a prophage produce a potent exotoxin that is absorbed in mucous membranes and causes remote damage to the liver, kidneys, and heart; the polypeptide toxin inhibits protein synthesis of the host cell. Although *C. diphtheriae* may infect the skin, it rarely invades the bloodstream and never actively invades deep tissue. Diphtheria toxin (DT) kills sensitive cells by blocking protein synthesis. DT is converted to an enzyme that inactivates EF-2, which is responsible for the translocation of polypeptidyl-tRNA from the acceptor to the donor site on the eukaryotic ribosome. The reaction is as follows:

$$NAD + EF\text{-}2 = ADP\text{-}ribosyl - EF\text{-}2 + nicotinamide + H^+$$

*B. pertussis* and *B. parapertussis* are similar and may be isolated together from a clinical specimen. However, *B. parapertussis* does not produce pertussis toxin. Pertussis toxin, like many bacterial toxins, has two subunits: A and B. Subunit A is an active enzyme, and B promotes binding of the toxin to host cells.

*F. tularensis* is a short, gram-negative organism that is markedly pleomorphic; it is nonmotile and cannot form spores. It has a rigid growth requirement for cysteine. Human tularemia usually is acquired from direct contact with tissues of infected rabbits but also can be transmitted by the bites of flies and ticks. *F. tularensis* causes a variety of clinical syndromes, including ulceroglandular, oculoglandular, pneumonic, and typhoidal forms of tularemia.

The pathogenesis of infection with *E. coli* is a complex interrelation of many events and properties. *E. coli* may serve as a model for other members of the Enterobacteriaceae. Some strains of *E. coli* are EIEC, some ETEC, some EHEC, and others EPEC. At the present time, there is little clinical significance in routinely discriminating the various types, with the possible exceptions of the ETEC and the *E. coli* 0157/H7 that are hemorrhagic. *E. coli* 0157/H7 secretes a toxin called *verotoxin*. The toxin is very active in a Vero cell line. More correctly, the toxin(s) should be called *Shiga-like*.

Streptococcal infection usually is accompanied by an elevated titer of antibody to some of the enzymes produced by the organism. Among the antigenic substances elaborated by group A β-hemolytic streptococci are erythrogenic toxin, streptodornase (streptococcal DNase), hyaluronidase, and streptolysin O (a hemolysin). Streptolysin S is a nonantigenic hemolysin. Specifically, erythrogenic toxin causes the characteristic rash of scarlet fever.

Many factors play a role in the pathogenesis of *N. meningitidis*. A capsule containing N-acetylneuraminic acid is peculiar to *Neisseria* and *E. coli* K1. Fresh isolates carry pili on their surfaces, which function in adhesion. *Neisseria* has a variety of membrane proteins, and their role in pathogenesis can only be speculated upon at this time. The lipopolysaccharide (LPS) of *Neisseria,* more correctly called lipooligosaccharide (LOS), is the endotoxic component of the cell.

There are no known toxins, hemolysins, or cell-wall constituents known to play a role in the pathogenesis of disease by *Brucella*. Rather, the ability of the organisms to survive within the host phagocyte and to inhibit neutrophil degranulation is a major disease-causing factor. In infectious abortion of cattle caused by *Brucella,* the tropism for placenta and the chorion is a function of the presence of erythritol in allantoic and amniotic fluid.

**285–289. The answers are 285-a, 286-b, 287-c, 288-b, 289-c.** *(Ryan, pp 851–855.)* "Atypical pneumonia" is an old classification used for respiratory disease that is not lobar and is not "typical." That is, it does not include pneumonia caused by pneumococcus, *Klebsiella, Haemophilus,* or β-hemolytic streptococci that results in a typical lobular infiltrate. In recent years, the atypical pneumonias have become much more frequent than pneumococcal pneumonia. They are characterized by a slower onset with headache, joint pain, fever, and signs of an acute upper respiratory infection. There are usually no signs of acute respiratory distress, but patients report malaise and fatigue. The most common cause of atypical pneumonia is *M. pneumoniae*. A quick test for *M. pneumoniae* infection is cold agglutinins. The test may lack both sensitivity and specificity, but it is rapid and readily available compared with culture of *M. pneumoniae* or specific antibody formation.

Particularly in the winter months, influenza must be ruled out. In the early stages of an epidemic, viral isolation in primary monkey cells is used. However, as the epidemic proceeds, diagnosis is usually made clinically or by an increase in antibody titer.

In certain age groups (men over 55 years old), Legionnaires' disease must be ruled out. While direct microscopy, culture, and serology are available, the detection of *Legionella* antigen in respiratory secretions is the most sensitive test available.

*C. pneumoniae* may also cause respiratory infection particularly in, but not limited to, children. Diagnosis is best made by growing these energy-defective bacteria in tissue culture such as HeLa cells. Serology is usually not helpful.

During the winter months, *Bordetella* infection may be quite prevalent, particularly in those patients whose immunizations are not current. Adult *Bordetella* infection may not present with typical whooping cough symptoms and must be differentiated from other forms of acute bronchitis by culture on specific media or direct fluorescent microscopy.

# Rickettsiae, Chlamydiae, and Mycoplasmas

## Questions

**DIRECTIONS:** Each question below contains four or more suggested responses. Select the **one best** response to each question.

**290.** Which of the following best describes the difference between mycoplasmas and chlamydiae?

a. Able to cause disease in humans
b. Able to cause urinary tract infection
c. Able to grow on artificial cell-free media
d. Able to stain well with Gram stain
e. Susceptible to penicillin

**291.** A 39-year-old man presents with sudden, influenza-like symptoms. He states that he works in a slaughterhouse, and several of his coworkers have similar symptoms. Early stages of pneumonia are detected. Which of the following is the most likely etiologic organism?

a. *Coxiella burnetti*
b. *Rickettsia ricketsiae*
c. *Taenia solium*
d. *Taenia saginata*

**292.** Which of the following best characterizes rickettsiae, which include the spotted fevers, Q fever, typhus, and scrub typhus?

a. Easily stained (gram-negative) with a Gram stain
b. Maintained in nature, with humans as the mammalian reservoir
c. Obligate intracellular parasites
d. Stable outside the host cell
e. The cause of infections in which a rash is always present

**293.** A man with chills, fever, and headache is thought to have "atypical" pneumonia. History reveals that he raises chickens, and that approximately 2 weeks ago he lost a large number of them to an undiagnosed disease. Which of the following is the most likely diagnosis of this man's condition?

a. Anthrax
b. Leptospirosis
c. Ornithosis
d. Relapsing fever
e. Q fever

**294.** An ill patient denies being bitten by insects. However, he spent some time in a milking barn and indicates that it was dusty. Of the following rickettsial diseases, which one has he most likely contracted?

a. Brill-Zinsser disease
b. Q fever
c. Rickettsialpox
d. Rocky Mountain spotted fever (RMSF)
e. Scrub typhus

**295.** A 23-year-old college senior presents to the student health clinic with symptoms of a suspected sexually transmitted disease (STD). *Neisseria* and *Chlamydia* agents are ruled out. Which of the following organisms is the most likely cause of his nongonococcal urethritis (NGU)?

a. *Mycoplasma fermentans*
b. *Mycoplasma hominis*
c. *Mycoplasma mycoides*
d. *Mycoplasma pneumoniae*
e. *Ureaplasma urealyticum*

**296.** A young man, home on leave from the military, went camping in the woods to detect deer movement for future hunting. Ten days later, he developed fever, malaise, and myalgia. Leukopenia and thrombocytopenia were observed, as well as several tick bites. Which of the following statements best describes human monocytic ehrlichiosis (HME)?

a. Clinical diagnosis is based on the presence of erythema migrans (EM)
b. Diagnosis is usually made serologically but morulae may be seen in the cytoplasm of monocytes
c. It is a fatal disease transmitted by the bite of a dog
d. Symptoms include vomiting and paralysis
e. The HME agent grows on artificial media

**297.** Lymphogranuloma venereum (LGV) is a venereal disease caused by serotype L1, L2, or L3 of *Chlamydia trachomatis*. The differential diagnosis should include which of the following?

a. Babesiosis
b. Chancroid
c. Mononucleosis
d. Psittacosis
e. Shingles

**298.** A forest worker experiences a sudden onset of fever, headache, myalgias, and prostration. A macular rash develops several days later, with it appearing first on the hands and feet before moving onto his trunk. Which of the following treatments is most appropriate?

a. Amphoteracin B
b. Cephalosporin
c. Erythromycin
d. Sulfonamides
e. Tetracycline

**299.** *C. trachomatis* can be distinguished from *Chlamydia psittaci* by which of the following criteria?

a. *C. psittaci* forms inclusions that contain glycogen
b. *C. psittaci* is an obligate prokaryotic parasite
c. *C. trachomatis* can be stained with Giemsa
d. *C. trachomatis* has a different lipopolysaccharide antigen
e. *C. trachomatis* is sensitive to sulfonamides

**300.** Chlamydiae have an unusual three-stage cycle of development. Which of the following is the correct sequence of these events?

a. Development of an initial body, synthesis of elementary body progeny, penetration of the host cell
b. Penetration of the host cell, development of an initial body, synthesis of elementary body progeny
c. Penetration of the host cell, synthesis of elementary body progeny, development of an initial body
d. Synthesis of elementary body progeny, development of an initial body, penetration of the host cell
e. Synthesis of elementary body progeny, penetration of the host cell, development of an initial body

**301.** Young children in a small Egyptian village had eye infections that presented with lacrimation, discharge, and conjunctival hyperemia. Scarring of the conjunctiva and noticeable loss of vision occurred in some. Which of the following statements best describes the etiologic agent which caused these infections and relative treatment?

a. The organisms are gram-positive and treatable with penicillin
b. The organisms have no cell wall and will only respond to tetracycline
c. The organisms are gram-negative, and prophylactic use of tetracyclines can prevent infections
d. Gram stains of conjunctival scrapings are useful diagnostic tests to justify treatment with sulfonamides
e. The organisms are isolated on blood agar plates and respond to cell-wall inhibiting antibiotics

**302.** Human granulocytic ehrlichiosis (HGE) is a disease transmitted to humans by the bite of a tick, *Ixodes scapularis*. Which of the following statements about HGE is correct?

a. Clinical diagnosis is based on the presence of EM
b. HGE is caused by *Ehrlichia chaffeensis*
c. HGE is a self-limiting disease
d. HGE is characterized by an acute onset of fever, severe headache, and influenza-like symptoms
e. The causative organism can be grown on ordinary laboratory media

**303.** The "spotted fever" group of rickettsial diseases is caused by a variety of rickettsial species. While not critical for treatment of disease, the speciation of these organisms is essential for epidemiologic studies. Which of the following rickettsiae is found in the United States and is a member of the spotted fever group?

a. *Rickettsia akari*
b. *Rickettsia australis*
c. *Rickettsia conorii*
d. *Rickettsia prowazekii*
e. *Rickettsia sibirica*

**304.** A 36-year-old man presents to his primary care physician's office complaining of fever and headache. On examination, he has leukopenia and increased liver enzymes, and inclusion bodies are seen in his monocytes. History reveals that he is outdoorsman and that he remembers removing a tick from his leg. Which of the following is the most likely diagnosis?

a. Ehrlichiosis
b. Lyme disease
c. Q fever
d. Rocky Mountain spotted fever
e. Tularemia

**305.** Typhus, spotted fever, and scrub typhus share which of the following manifestations of disease?

a. Arthritis
b. Common vector
c. Fever and rash
d. Short incubation period (<48 h)
e. Similar geographic distribution

**306.** *C. trachomatis* is a well-known cause of venereal disease. This organism is also implicated in which of the following?

a. Blindness
b. Middle-ear infection in young children
c. Perinatal retinitis
d. Sexually transmitted cardiac disease in adults
e. Urinary tract infection in children

**307.** A homosexual male presents to his physician with bilateral inguinal buboes (lymph nodes), one of which seems ready to rupture. He recalls having two small, painless genital lesions that healed rapidly. The etiologic agent is isolated using McCoy cells. Which of the following statements best characterizes LGV?

a. It is most common in temperate regions
b. In the United States, it is more common among women
c. The causative agent is *C. trachomatis*
d. The disease (LGV) does not become chronic
e. Penicillin is effective in early treatment

**308.** Dozens of political refugees fleeing from active warfare and living in a dense forest environment with crowded, unsanitary conditions experienced nonspecific symptoms, followed by high fever and severe headache, along with chills, myalgia, and arthralgia. All had body lice. Improved living conditions in a refugee camp and treatment with tetracycline brought resolution to most individuals. Which of the following statements describes the etiological agent responsible for their infection?

a. The disease was caused by an organism with no cell walls
b. The disease was caused by a viral agent
c. The disease was derived from rodents living in the forest area
d. Reoccurrence of milder disease may occur in later years
e. The disease was caused by a tick vector

**309.** Chlamydiae are small, gram-negative rods once thought to be viruses. Which of the following best characterizes chlamydiae as distinct from viruses?

a. Cannot visualize with light microscope
b. Independent synthesis of proteins
c. Intracellular reproduction
d. Susceptibility to antimicrobial agents (penicillins)
e. Synthesis of ATP

**310.** *Chlamydia pneumoniae*, sometimes known as *Chlamydia* "TWAR," is the most recent *Chlamydia* species to be associated with human disease. Which one of the following statements best describes *C. pneumoniae?*

a. *C. pneumoniae* has been associated with myocardial infarction
b. *C. pneumoniae* infections are generally severe
c. *C. pneumoniae* infections are uncommon—up to 10% of adults may show specific antibody
d. Infections with *C. pneumoniae* usually arise from bacterial overgrowth in the colon
e. Nonpsittacine birds are reservoirs of *C. pneumoniae*

**311.** Primary atypical pneumonia (PAP) is generally a mild disease, ranging from subclinical infection to serious pneumonitis, the latter characterized by onset of fever, headache, sore throat, and cough. Which of the following organisms causes this disease in humans?

a. *M. fermentans*
b. *M. hominis*
c. *M. pneumoniae*
d. *Mycoplasma orale*
e. *U. urealyticum*

**312.** While the majority of NGU are caused by *Chlamydiae trachomatis*, which of the following organisms is very significant in causing additional cases in humans?

a. *M. fermentans*
b. *M. hominis*
c. *M. pneumoniae*
d. *M. orale*
e. *U. urealyticum*

**313.** A healthy oral cavity has a microbial population consisting of gram-positive streptococci and diphtheroids. Anaerobic rods and spirochetes are present in low numbers and may be opportunistic for disease. Which of the following organisms also normally inhabits the healthy human oral cavity?

a. *M. fermentans*
b. *M. hominis*
c. *M. pneumoniae*
d. *M. orale*
e. *U. urealyticum*

**314.** Which of the following organisms normally inhabits the female genital tract but may cause acute respiratory illness?

a.  *M. fermentans*
b.  *M. hominis*
c.  *M. pneumoniae*
d.  *M. orale*
e.  *U. urealyticum*

**315.** Which of the following is the causative agent that is sexually transmitted and characterized by suppurative inguinal adenitis?

a.  *Bartonella (Rochalimaea) henselae*
b.  *C. trachomatis*
c.  *Coxsiella burnetii*
d.  *E. chaffeensis*
e.  *Rickettsia rickettsii*

**316.** Which of the following is transmitted by the bite of a hard *Ixodes* tick and is treatable with tetracycline?

a.  *Bartonella (Rochalimaea) henselae*
b.  *C. trachomatis*
c.  *Coxsiella burnetii*
d.  *E. chaffeensis*
e.  *R. rickettsii*

**317.** Cat-scratch disease is usually a benign, self-limited illness manifested by fever and lymphadenopathy that develops about 2 weeks after contact with a cat. Which of the following microorganisms is the causative agent of this infection?

a.  *B. (Rochalimaea) henselae*
b.  *C. trachomatis*
c.  *C. burnetii*
d.  *E. chaffeensis*
e.  *R. rickettsii*

**318.** Which of the following is a gram-negative bacteria with tropism for mononuclear cells and may cause infections via the respiratory pathway?

a. *B. (Rochalimaea) henselae*
b. *C. trachomatis*
c. *C. burnetii*
d. *E. chaffeensis*
e. *R. rickettsii*

**319.** Which of the following is the etiologic agent of a disease found in the Western Hemisphere, is transmitted by tick bites, and may exhibit a wide range of systemic manifestations?

a. *B. (Rochalimaea) henselae*
b. *C. trachomatis*
c. *C. burnetii*
d. *E. chaffeensis*
e. *R. rickettsii*

# Rickettsiae, Chlamydiae, and Mycoplasmas

## Answers

**290. The answer is c.** *(Brooks, pp 343–347. Levinson, pp 166–167, 173–175. Murray—2005, pp 444–446. Ryan, pp 409, 463.)* Unlike the chlamydiae, they can replicate in cell-free media. Mycoplasmas lack a rigid cell wall and are bound by a triple-layer unit membrane. For this reason, they are completely resistant to the action of penicillins.

**291. The answer is a.** *(Brooks, pp 349–356. Levinson, pp 176–178. Murray—2005, pp 449–460. Ryan, p 477.)* Q fever is an acute, flulike illness caused by *C. burnetii*. It is the one rickettsial disease not transmitted by the bite of a tick. *C. burnetii* is found in high concentrations in the urine, feces, and placental tissue/amniotic fluid of cattle, goats, and sheep. Transmission to humans is by aerosol inhalation of those specimens. *R. rickettsiae* is present in the US and South America, but is transmitted by ticks that feed on rodents or dogs. The parasitic *Taenia* species are transmitted by ingestion of undercooked meat.

**292. The answer is c.** *(Brooks, pp 349–356. Levinson, pp 176–178. Murray—2005, pp 449–460. Ryan, pp 472–473.)* Rickettsiae are obligate intracellular parasites that depend on host cells for their phosphorylated energy compounds. The significant rickettsial diseases in North America include RMSF (*R. rickettsii*), Q fever (*Coxiella burnetii*), and typhus (*R. prowazekii*, *Rickettsia typhi*). Laboratory diagnosis of rickettsial disease is based on serologic analysis rather than isolation of the organism.

**293. The answer is c.** *(Brooks, pp 357–365. Levinson, pp 173–175. Murray—2005, pp 463–472. Ryan, p 469.)* Ornithosis (psittacosis) is caused by *C. psittaci*. Humans usually contract the disease from infected birds kept as pets or from infected poultry, including poultry in dressing plants. Although ornithosis may be asymptomatic in humans, severe pneumonia can develop. Fortunately, the disease is cured easily with tetracycline.

**294. The answer is b.** *(Brooks, pp 349–356. Levinson, pp 176–178. Murray—2005, pp 449–460. Ryan, p 477.)* Most rickettsial diseases are transmitted to humans by way of arthropod vectors. The only exception is Q fever, which is caused by *Coxiella burnetii.* This organism is transmitted by inhalation of contaminated dust and aerosols or by ingestion of contaminated milk.

**295. The answer is e.** *(Brooks, pp 343–346. Levinson, pp 166–167. Murray—2005, pp 443–448. Ryan, p 413.)* U. urealyticum has been associated with NGU as well as infertility. *M. pneumoniae* is the etiologic agent of PAP. *M. hominis,* although isolated from up to 30% of patients with NGU, has yet to be implicated as a cause of that disease. *M. fermentans* has on rare occasions been isolated from the oropharynx and genital tract. *M. mycoides* causes bovine pleuropneumonia.

**296. The answer is b.** *(Brooks, pp 349–356. Levinson, p 167. Murray—2005, pp 449–460. Ryan, p 478.)* HME, caused by the bite of the tick *Amblyomma americanum* infected with *E. chaffeensis,* causes an illness not unlike RMSF, except a rash usually does not occur. Diagnosis is usually made serologically, and treatment of choice is tetracycline. Symptoms include high fever, severe headache, and myalgias.

**297. The answer is b.** *(Brooks, pp 360–362. Levinson, pp 168–172. Murray—2005, pp 363–372. Ryan, pp 466–467.)* The differential diagnosis of LGV includes syphilis, genital herpes, and chancroid. Several clinical tests can be used to rule out syphilis and genital herpes. These include a negative (negative to rule out; positive to rule in) dark-field examination as well as positive serologic findings for syphilis and the demonstration of herpes simplex virus by cytology or culture. *Haemophilus ducreyi* can usually be isolated from the ulcer in chancroid.

**298. The answer is e.** *(Brooks, pp 360–365. Levinson, pp 176–178. Murray—2005, pp 469–470. Ryan, p 475.)* Tetracyclines and chloramphenicol are effective, provided treatment is started early for rickettsial diseases, including RMSF, as in this case. Those should be given orally daily and continued for several days after the rash subsides. IV dosage can be used in severely ill patients. Sulfonamides enhance the disease and are contraindicated. The other antibiotics are ineffective. Antibiotics only suppress the bacteria's growth, and the patient's immune system must eradicate them.

**299. The answer is e.** *(Brooks, p 359. Levinson, pp 173–175. Murray—2005, p 469. Ryan, p 463.)* The chlamydiae are obligate prokaryotic parasites of eukaryotic cells. For many years, they were considered to be viruses but are now considered to be bacteria. The two species, *C. trachomatis* and *C. psittaci*, can be distinguished by two criteria: the susceptibility of *C. trachomatis* to sulfonamides and its ability to form inclusions containing glycogen. Chlamydiae are obligate intracellular bacteria and are seen using Giemsa staining.

**300. The answer is b.** *(Brooks, p 357. Levinson, pp 173–175. Murray—2005, p 465. Ryan, p 465.)* The developmental cycle of chlamydiae begins with the elementary body attaching to and then penetrating the host cell. The elementary body, now in a vacuole bounded by host-cell membrane, becomes an initial body. Within about 12 hours, the initial body has divided to form many small elementary particles encased within an inclusion body in the cytoplasm; these progeny are liberated by host-cell rupture.

**301. The answer is c.** *(Brooks, pp 357–366. Levinson, pp 173–175. Murray—2005, pp 464–468. Ryan, pp 464–466.)* C. trachomatis serovars A, B, Ba, and C are responsible for endemic trachoma. While diagnosis is usually dependent upon observation of intracellular inclusions with a glycogen matrix in which elementary bodies are embedded, Gram stain preparations are not useful diagnostic tools. The cell wall most closely resembles a gram high lipid content and may stain gram-negative or variable. A single monthly dose of doxycycline can result in significant clinical improvement and be preventative.

**302. The answer is d.** *(Brooks, pp 350–354. Levinson, pp 180–181, 484s. Murray—2005, pp 458–459. Ryan, p 478.)* HGE is caused by the bite of *I. scapularis* infected with either *Ehrlichia phagocytophilia* or *Ehrlichia ewingii* or *Echichia equi* (Levinson, p 181, 8th ed.). A rash rarely occurs and EM does not occur, but the symptoms (fever, chills, headache, myalgia, nausea, vomiting, anorexia, and weight loss) are similar to those seen in RMSF. Serological tests show that subclinical ehrlichiosis occurs frequently.

**303. The answer is a.** *(Brooks, pp 349–356. Levinson, p 163. Murray—2005, pp 449–456. Ryan, p 473.)* The primary cause of RMSF is *R. rickettsii*, although rickettsialpox is caused by *R. akari*, the only other member of the spotted fever group that resides in the United States. *R. sibirica* is responsible for tick typhus in China; *R. australis* causes typhus in Australia, as the name signifies; and *R. conorii* causes European and African rickettsioses. *R. prowazekii* is not a member of the spotted fever group; it causes epidemic typhus.

**304. The answer is a.** *(Brooks, pp 349–356. Levinson, pp 168–172, 180–181, 484s. Murray—2005, pp 449–456. Ryan, p 478.)* All the listed diseases except Q fever are tick-borne. The rickettsia *C. burnetii* causes Q fever, and humans are usually infected by aerosol of a sporelike form shed in milk, urine, feces, or placenta of infected sheep, cattle, or goats. Lyme disease is caused by a spirochete, *Borrelia burgdorferi*, and produces the characteristic lesion erythema chronicum migrans (ECM). The etiologic agent of RMSF is *R. rickettsia.* It usually produces a rash that begins in the extremities and then involves the trunk. Two human forms of ehrlichiosis can occur: HME, caused by *E. chaffeensis,* and HGE, caused by an as yet unnamed *Ehrlichia.* Ehrlichiosis was previously recognized only as a veterinary pathogen. HME infection is transmitted by the brown dog tick and *A. americanum.* HGE infection is transmitted by *I. scapularis,* the same tick that transmits Lyme disease. Both infections cause fever and leukopenia. A rash rarely occurs. *E. chaffeensis* infects monocytes, and HGE infects granulocytes; both organisms produce inclusion bodies called *morulae. Francisella tularensis* is a small, gram-negative, nonmotile coccobacillus. Humans most commonly acquire the organism after contact with the tissues or body fluid of an infected mammal or the bite of an infected tick.

**305. The answer is c.** *(Brooks, pp 349–356. Levinson, pp 176–178. Murray— 2005, pp 449–456. Ryan, pp 473–475.)* Typhus, spotted fever, and scrub typhus are all caused by rickettsiae (*R. prowazekii, R. rickettsii,* and *Rickettsia tsutsugamushi,* respectively). Clinically, the diseases have several similarities. Each has an incubation period of 1–2 weeks, followed by a febrile period, which usually includes a rash. During the febrile period, rickettsiae can be found in the patient's blood, and there is disseminated focal vasculitis of small blood vessels. The geographic area associated with these diseases is usually different. Scrub typhus is usually found in Japan, Southeast Asia, and the Pacific, while spotted fever is usually found in the Western hemisphere. Typhus has a worldwide incidence. (Typhus—lice and fleas, spotted fever—ticks and mites, scrub—mites.)

**306. The answer is a.** *(Brooks, pp 357–362. Levinson, pp 173–175. Murray—2005, pp 463–472. Ryan, p 464.)* Trachoma has been the greatest single cause of blindness in the world. *C. trachomatis* is the most common cause of STD in the United States and is also responsible for the majority of cases of infant conjunctivitis and infant pneumonia.

**307. The answer is c.** *(Brooks, pp 360–362. Levinson, pp 173–175. Murray—2005, pp 463–472. Ryan, pp 466–468.)* LGV is a STD caused by *C. trachomatis* of immunotypes L1, L2, and L3. It is more commonly found in tropical climates. In the United States, the sex ratio is reported to be 3.4 males to 1 female. Tetracycline has been successful in treating this disease in the early stages; however, late stages usually require surgery.

**308. The answer is d.** *(Brooks, pp 349–356. Levinson, pp 176–178. Murray—2005, pp 449–456. Ryan, pp 475–476.)* The disease described is epidemic typhus or louse-borne typhus. It is caused by *R. prowazekii* and is spread by the human body louse, *Pediculus humanus.* Lice obviously occur most readily in unsanitary conditions brought on by war or natural disasters, where normal healthy living conditions are unavailable. Rickettsial diseases respond to tetracycline treatment and vector control. The organisms replicate in endothelial cells, resulting in vasculitis. Recrudescent disease (recurrence in later years) has been demonstrated in people exposed to epidemic typhus during World War II. This form of disease is generally milder, and convalescence is shorter.

**309. The answer is b.** *(Brooks, pp 357–360. Levinson, pp 173–175. Murray—2005, pp 463–472. Ryan, pp 463–464.)* Although both chlamydiae and viruses are obligate, intracellular parasites and depend on the host cell for ATP and phosphorylated intermediates, they differ in many respects. Unlike viruses, chlamydiae synthesize proteins and reproduce by fission. Chlamydiae are readily seen under the light microscope and possess bacteria-like cell walls.

**310. The answer is a.** *(Brooks, p 363. Levinson, pp 173–175. Murray—2005, pp 463–472. Ryan, p 470.)* A distinct group of chlamydiae, first designated "TWAR," has been given the name *C. pneumoniae.* The strain was first isolated in Taiwan and usually causes mild acute respiratory disease. *C. psittaci* causes a respiratory syndrome and is associated with avian contact. *C. pneumoniae* has no avian vector. Recent evidence suggests that *C. pneumoniae* may be involved in cardiac disease, possibly as part of an autoimmune phenomenon. This organism has recently had a genus name change to *Chlamydophila*.

**311–314. The answers are 311-c, 312-e, 313-d, 314-b.** *(Brooks, pp 343–348. Levinson, pp 166–167. Murray—2005, pp 443–448. Ryan, pp 409–412.)* Members of the mycoplasma group that are pathogenic for humans include *M. pneumoniae* and *U. urealyticum*. *M. pneumoniae* is best known as the causative agent of PAP, which may be confused clinically with influenza or legionellosis. It also is associated with arthritis, pericarditis, aseptic meningitis, and the Guillain-Barré syndrome. *M. pneumoniae* can be cultivated on special media and identified by immunofluorescence staining and "fried egg" colonies on agar.

*U. urealyticum* (once called *tiny*, or *T, strain*) has been implicated in cases of NGU. As the name implies, this organism is able to split urea, a fact of diagnostic significance. *U. urealyticum* is part of the normal flora of the genitourinary tract, particularly in women.

Both *M. orale* and *Mycoplasma salivarium* are inhabitants of the normal human oral cavity. These species are commensals and do not play a role in disease.

The only other species of *Mycoplasma* associated with human disease is *M. hominis*. A normal inhabitant of the genital tract of women, this organism has been demonstrated to produce an acute respiratory illness that is associated with sore throat and tonsillar exudate, but not with fever.

*M. fermentans* is an animal isolate.

**315–319. The answers are 315-b, 316-d, 317-a, 318-c, 319-e.** *(Brooks, pp 349–356, 357–366. Levinson, pp 173–175, 180–181, 176–178. Murray— 2005, pp 449–456, 463–472. Ryan, pp 463–470, 471–479.)* Rickettsiae are small bacteria that are obligate, intracellular parasites. Most but not all rickettsiae are transmitted to humans by arthropods. *Coxiella* is transmitted through the respiratory tract rather than through the skin, and *B. henselae* from animal scratches. *Coxiella* may cause chronic endocarditis that is not very responsive to either antimicrobial therapy or valve replacement. *B. henselae* is a fastidious, gram-negative rod that causes bacillary angiomatosis, a disease that forms dermal or subcutaneous nodules. The role of *B. henselae* in cat-scratch disease has recently been recognized. Molecular taxonomic studies have indicated that the causative organism is more closely related to *Bartonella* than to *Rochalimaea*, hence the name change.

*Ehrlichia* is an obligate, intracellular parasite that resembles rickettsia. *E. chaffeensis* has been linked to human ehrlichiosis, although this infection is primarily seen in animals. The majority of patients with this disease report exposure to ticks. It is thought that *I. scapularis* carries *Ehrlichia*, although the Lone Star tick, *A. americanum*, may also transmit the disease.

Chlamydiae are gram-negative bacteria that are obligate, intracellular parasites. They are divided into three species: *C. trachomatis, C. pneumoniae,* and *C. psittaci.* Chlamydiae have a unique developmental cycle. The infectious particle is the elementary body. Once inside the cell, the elementary body undergoes reorganization to form a reticulate body. After several replications, the reticulate bodies differentiate into elementary bodies, are released from the host cell, and become available to infect other cells. Three of the 15 serovars of *C. trachomatis* (L1, L2, L3) are known to cause LGV, a STD. *C. trachomatis* is a leading cause of STD in the United States. It is insidious because so many early infections are asymptomatic, particularly in women.

RMSF is a spotted fever caused by *R. rickettsii* and is characterized by acute onset of fever, severe headache, and myalgias. The rash occurs 2–6 days later, first in the hands and feet, and then moves to the trunk. Diagnosis must be made on clinical presentations, and therapy instituted immediately. Laboratory diagnosis is made on a rising antibody titer (delayed). Untreated disease can be fatal.

# Mycology

## Questions

**320.** A leukemic patient complains of respiratory symptoms including frequent coughs. An examination of the left lung reveals the presence of a coin-sized lesion characterized by the presence of an air space surrounding the cavity. Sputa of the patient show the presence of a thick, uniformly septate hyphae. The culture yields hairy colonies firmly adhering to the medium surface. The patient is tuberculin negative. Which of the following is the most likely cause of the respiratory problem in this patient?

a. Aspergillosis
b. Candidiasis
c. Histoplasmosis
d. Mucormycosis
e. Tuberculosis

**321.** A 62-year-old white male is admitted to the hospital complaining of shortness of breath. His medical history indicates he has smoked 1 pack of cigarettes per day for the past 40 years. Recently, he has been on immuno-suppressive therapy for severe arthritis. A biopsy specimen of the lung is obtained, and septate hyphae that form V-shaped branches are observed. Culture on agar shows conidia with spores in radiating columns (see the figure). Which of the following is consistent with these diagnostic findings?

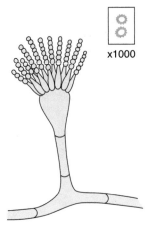

x1000

(Reproduced, with permission, from Brooks GF et al. Jawetz's Medical Microbiology, 22e. New York: McGraw-Hill, 2001: 534.)

a. Aspergillosis
b. Emphysema
c. Lung cancer
d. *Pneumocystis carinii* pneumonia
e. Viral pneumonia
f. Zygomycosis

**322.** The object designated by the arrow in the following photomicrograph is which of the following?

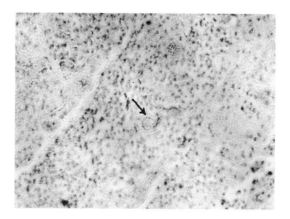

a.  An encapsulated yeast
b.  A hyphal strand
c.  A macroconidium
d.  A spherule
e.  A thick-walled spore

**323.** A 6-year-old girl presents to the clinic with scaly patches on the scalp. Primary smears and culture of the skin and hair are negative. A few weeks later, she returns and is found to have inflammatory lesions. The hair fluoresces under Wood's light, and primary smears of skin and hair contain septate hyphae. On speaking with the parents, it is discovered that there are several pets in the household. Which of the following is the most likely infecting agent?

a.  *Epidermophyton floccosum*
b.  *Microsporum audouinii*
c.  *Microsporum canis*
d.  *Trichophyton rubrum*
e.  *Trichophyton tonsurans*

**324.** A patient with AIDS has a persistent cough and has shown progressive behavioral changes in the past few weeks after eating an under-cooked hamburger. A cerebrospinal fluid (CSF) sample is collected and an encapsulated, yeastlike organism is observed. Based only on these observations, which of the following is the most likely organism?

a. *Candida*
b. *Cryptococcus*
c. *Cryptosporidium*
d. *Pneumocystis*
e. *Toxoplasma*

**325.** A chronically ill, young, white male is unable to work due to his frequent illnesses. He spends most of his time raising and training pigeons. He develops a mild pulmonary infection and eventually presents to his primary care physician with headache, mental status changes, and fever. A clinical diagnosis of meningitis is confirmed with a latex agglutination test on CSF for the capsular polysaccharide of the organism. Which of the following is the most likely causative agent?

a. *Aspergillus fumigatus*
b. *Candida albicans*
c. *Cryptococcus neoformans*
d. *Histoplasma capsulatum*
e. *Paracoccidioides brasiliensis*

**326.** A section of tissue from the foot of a person assumed to have eumycotic mycetoma shows a white, lobulated granule composed of fungal hyphae. In the United States, the most common etiologic agent of this condition is a species of which of the following?

a. *Acremonium*
b. *Actinomyces*
c. *Madurella*
d. *Nocardia*
e. *Pseudallescheria*

**327.** A healthy middle-aged construction worker who engaged in a demolition task 10 days earlier complains of respiratory symptoms similar to those of pneumonia. No causative agent has been isolated from his sputa. The patient does not respond to any antibacterial antibiotics and dies before a definitive diagnosis was established. Microscopic examination of specimens taken of granulomatous and suppurative lesions of the lung obtained during necropsy reveal the presence of large budding yeast cells. The bud is attached to the parent cell by a broad base. Based on this information, which of the following is the most likely diagnosis?

a. Blastomycosis
b. Coccidioidomycosis
c. Cryptococcosis
d. Histoplasmosis
e. Sporotrichosis

**328.** Infection with *Sporothrix schenckii* (formerly *Sporotrichum schenckii*) is an occupational hazard for gardeners. The portal of entry for this organism is via which of the following routes?

a. Lymphatic system
b. Mouth
c. Mucous membranes
d. Respiratory tract
e. Skin

**329.** There are three genera of dermatophytes: *Epidermophyton, Microsporum,* and *Trichophyton.* Which of the following statements characterizes the infections caused by these organisms?

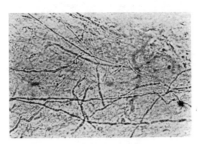

*(Courtesy of MG Rinaldi, San Antonio, TX)*

a.  Characterized by aflatoxin-induced hallucinations
b.  Confined to keratinized tissues
c.  Easily treatable with penicillin
d.  Marked by alveolar irritation
e.  Rarely associated with chronic lesions

**330.** A 57-year-old obese white female is referred to your clinic due to a sore throat characterized by a white pseudomembranous lesion of epithelial cells and organisms. The patient's history reveals type 1 diabetes mellitus and recent penicillin use for a severe bacterial infection in her right foot. Which of the following will most likely be present on microscopic examination?

a.  Abundance of septate rhizoids
b.  Asci containing 2–8 ascospores
c.  Metachromatic granules
d.  Spherules containing endospores
e.  Yeasts and pseudohyphae

**331.** The mechanism of mucosal invasion by *C. albicans* is at least partially understood. Which of the following modifications in the structure or function of this yeast is most likely to affect its invasive ability?

a.  Loss of ability to produce ethanol from glucose
b.  Loss of ability to produce germ tubes or hyphae
c.  Loss of ability to produce a polysaccharide capsule
d.  Reduced ability to grow at 37°C
e.  Replacement of mannans in the cell wall with glucan

**332.** You have been designated as coordinator of construction of a bone marrow transplant unit (BMTU). There will be extensive removal of walls and floors in order to install the laminar flow rooms required for a BMTU. From the standpoint of frequency and lethality, which of the following fungi should be your biggest concern?

a. *Aspergillus*
b. *Blastomyces*
c. *Candida*
d. *Cryptococcus*
e. *Wangiella*

**333.** *H. capsulatum,* a dimorphic fungus, is found in soil heavily contaminated with bird droppings. Which of the following statements best describes the presence of the organism in tissue biopsies?

a. Arthrospores
b. Oval budding yeasts inside macrophages
c. Single-cell yeasts with pseudohyphae
d. Spherules containing endospores
e. Yeasts with broad-based bud

**334.** A 65-year-old female patient is admitted to an intensive care unit because of sudden swelling on the right side of the face and an episode of bleeding from the right nostril. According to her daughter, these signs were not apparent a few days ago. She has a long history of diabetes, high blood pressure, and recently developed clinical signs of ketoacidosis and renal insufficiency. Her blood sugar level at the time of admission is 700 mg/dL. The facial lesion becomes partially necrotic and shows slight protursion of the right eye and facial paralysis. The patient dies on the second day. Histopathologic examination of the lesions reveals occlusion of the small vessels and the presence of nonseptate hyphae. This is most probably caused by which of the following?

a. Candadiasis
b. Erysipelis
c. Gas gangrene
d. Mucormycosis
e. Nocardiosis

**335.** Inhalation of fungal spores can cause primary lung infections. Which of the following organisms is associated with this mode of transmission?

a. *C. albicans*
b. *Candida tropicalis*
c. *C. immitis*
d. *S. schenckii*
e. *T. tonsurans*

**336.** An immunocompromised patient is suspected of having an infection with *A. fumigatus*. Which of the following clinical conditions is most likely to occur?

a. Invasive infection causing thrombosis and infarction
b. Superficial rash
c. Thrush
d. Urinary tract infection
e. Wound infection

**337.** A 25-year-old pregnant woman, living in the San Joaquin Valley (California) experienced an influenza-like illness with fever and cough. She was diagnosed with *Coccidioides* infection that disseminated from her lungs to other organs while in the third trimester of pregnancy. Patients who have disseminated coccidioidomycosis usually demonstrate which of the following?

a. Absence of complement-fixing (CF) antibodies
b. A negative coccidioidin skin test and a rising CF titer
c. A negative coccidioidin skin test and a stable CF titer
d. A positive skin test and a mildly elevated CF titer
e. Lack of immunity to reinfection

**338.**  *C. albicans* (shown in the figure) is best described by which of the following statements?

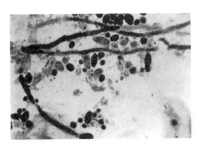

*Candida albicans.* Yeast cells (blastoconidia) and pseudohyphae in exudate. *(Reproduced, with permission, from Brooks GF et al. Jawetz's Medical Microbiology, 23e. New York: McGraw-Hill, 2004:646.)*

a. Round, black sporangia filled with endospores; sporangia unbranched, rising from a runner called a stolon
b. Single-tipped sporangiophores; no rhizoids or stolons; nonseptate hyphae, which show branching
c. Widespread in environment; conidia may be inhaled; microscopic appearance in specimen reveals dichotomous branching and septate hyphae
d. Yeast forms with budding blastoconidia often showing pseudohyphae; positive germ tube test; chlamydospores present

**339.**  *Aspergillus* is best described by which of the following statements?

a. Round, black sporangia filled with endospores; sporangia unbranched, rising from a runner called a stolon
b. Single-tipped sporangiophores; no rhizoids or stolons; nonseptate hyphae, which show branching
c. Widespread in environment; conidia may be inhaled; microscopic appearance in specimen reveals dichotomous branching and septate hyphae
d. Yeast forms with budding blastoconidia often showing pseudohyphae; positive germ tube test; chlamydospores present

**340.** *Mucor* is best described by which of the following statements?

a. Round, black sporangia filled with endospores; sporangia unbranched, rising from a runner called a stolon
b. Single-tipped sporangiophores; no rhizoids or stolons; nonseptate hyphae, which show branching
c. Widespread in environment; conidia may be inhaled; microscopic appearance in specimen reveals dichotomous branching and septate hyphae
d. Yeast forms with budding blastoconidia often showing pseudohyphae; positive germ tube test; chlamydospores present

**341.** *Rhizopus* is best described by which of the following statements?

a. Round, black sporangia filled with endospores; sporangia unbranched, rising from a runner called a stolon
b. Single-tipped sporangiophores; no rhizoids or stolons; nonseptate hyphae, which show branching
c. Widespread in environment; conidia may be inhaled; microscopic appearance in specimen reveals dichotomous branching and septate hyphae
d. Yeast forms with budding blastoconidia often showing pseudohyphae; positive germ tube test; chlamydospores present

**342.** A 37-year-old Asian male is admitted to the hospital complaining of shortness of breath. He denies use of cigarettes, although he admits a previous history of intravenous drug abuse. His chest films show a diffuse ground glass pattern. A specimen is obtained by bronchoalveolar lavage, and distinctive thin-walled trophozoites and thick-walled spherical cysts containing 4–8 nucleii are observed using methenamine-silver stain. Which of the following is the most likely diagnosis?

a. AIDS-related lymphoma
b. Aspergillosis
c. Blastomycosis
d. Histoplasmosis
e. *P. carinii* pneumonia

**343.** An 18-year-old white male high-school student visited the school nurses' office complaining of a diffuse, painful rash extending from his midthigh to his navel region. He indicates that one of his football team-mates gave him topical hydrocortisone to initially treat a minor groin rash. A KOH scraping of the lesion revealed the organisms shown in the figure. Which of the following is the most likely diagnosis?

*Epidermophyton floccosum*

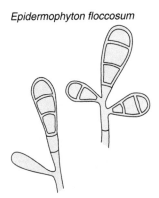

(*Reproduced, with permission, from Brooks GF et al. Jawetz's Medical Microbiology, 22e. New York: McGraw-Hill, 2001:536.*)

a. Coccidioidomycosis
b. Herpes simplex infection
c. Herpes zoster infection
d. Secondary syphilis
e. Tinea corporis (incognito)

**344.** A medical student was serving as a missionary in Africa. While assisting with the construction of a water project, a thorn pierced the glove of his left hand. Several days after the inflammation from the initial wound subsided, necrotizing lesions began to form that spread toward the elbow. Which of the following is the most likely etiological agent?

a. *C. immitis*
b. *Malassezia furfur*
c. *M. canis*
d. *S. schenkii*
e. *Stachybotrys chartarum*

**345.** A 30-year-old patient was generally healthy until his impacted wisdom tooth was removed by an oral surgeon. The area where the tooth had been was sore, but what was more alarming was the appearance of eruptions through the skin beneath the area of the jaw where the tooth had been. The exudate draining through the skin eruptions was cultured aerobically, but the results were negative. Which of the following is the most likely etiologic agent responsible for the patient's condition?

a. *Actinomyces bovis*
b. *Actinomyces israelii*
c. *C. albicans*
d. *H. capsulatum*
e. *Nocardia asteroides*

**346.** Several laboratory tests were researched for their usefulness in evaluating suspected histoplasmosis in patients who reside in an area where the disease is endemic. If the prevalence of histoplasmosis is 25%, which of the following sensitivity and specificity combinations would be the most useful confirmatory test for diagnosing the disease?

a. Sensitivity of 50%, specificity of 98%
b. Sensitivity of 90%, specificity of 80%
c. Sensitivity of 92%, specificity of 70%
d. Sensitivity of 99%, specificity of 90%

**347.** Which of the following is associated with *H. capsulatum?*

a. Arthroconidia
b. Sclerotic bodies
c. Spherules
d. Tuberculate macroconidia

**348.** Individuals taking broad-spectrum antibiotics such as tetracycline often develop candidiasis. Which of the following statements is true?

a. The antibiotic enhances the growth of *C. albicans.*
b. Tetracycline is known to inhibit ergosterol synthesis.
c. Broad-spectrum antibiotics upset the balance of normal microbial flora.
d. The antibiotic damages the host oral epithelium.
e. Tetracycline drastically increases DNA synthesis by *C. albicans.*

**349.** Valley fever or desert rheumatism is asymptomatic in 60% of individuals, while 40% present with a self limited influenza-like illness with fever, malaise, cough, arthralgia, and headache. Less than 1% develop life-threatening CNS complications. The highly infectious asexual conidia of the etiologic agent are called which of the following?

a. Arthroconidia
b. Blastoconidia
c. Chlamydospores
d. Sporangiospores

**350.** Tinea corporis is caused by which of the following?

a. *E. floccosum*
b. *Exophiala werneckii*
c. *M. furfur*
d. *M. canis*
e. *Trichosporon beigelii*

**351.** Tinea pedis is caused by which of the following?

a. *E. floccosum*
b. *E. werneckii*
c. *M. furfur*
d. *M. canis*
e. *T. beigelii*

**352.** Tinea capitis is caused by which of the following?

a. *E. floccosum*
b. *E. werneckii*
c. *M. furfur*
d. *M. canis*
e. *T. beigelii*

**353.** Tinea versicolor is caused by which of the following?

a. *E. floccosum*
b. *E. werneckii*
c. *M. furfur*
d. *M. canis*
e. *T. beigelii*

**354.** A young man in his mid-twenties presents with mucosal lesions in his mouth. Based on his CD4 cell count and other signs during the past few months, he is diagnosed as having AIDS. Which of the following is the most likely etiology of the oral lesions?

a. *Aspergillus*
b. *Candida*
c. *Cryptococcus*
d. *Mucor*
e. *Rhizopus*

**355.** It is difficult to determine whether isolation from one body site or body fluid is suggestive of colonization or infection. Which of the following fungi is often isolated from blood, urine, and sputum in invasive disease?

a. *A. fumigatus*
b. *Basidiobolus ranarum*
c. *C. albicans*
d. *Conidiobolus coronata*
e. *Rhizopus arrhizus*

**356.** Which of the following fungi causes rhinocerebral zygomycosis and is usually associated with acute diabetes?

a. *A. fumigatus*
b. *B. ranarum*
c. *C. albicans*
d. *C. coronata*
e. *R. arrhizus*

**357.** Three weeks after a patient with AIDS traveled to California to study desert flowers, he develops fever, chest pain, and muscle soreness. Two months later, red, tender nodules appear on the shins, and he has pain and tenderness in the right ankle. An x-ray film of the chest shows a left pleural effusion. Which of the following is the most likely diagnosis?

a. Blastomycosis
b. Coccidioidomycosis
c. Histoplasmosis
d. *Mycobacterium marinum* infection
e. *Mycoplasma pneumoniae* infection

**358.** Which of the following fungi resides in the soil and is introduced into the skin by traumatic inoculation of contaminated material?

a. A. fumigatus
b. Coccidioides immitis
c. C. neoformans
d. H. capsulatum
e. S. schenckii

**359.** An 18-year-old high school student in rural north Mississippi develops fever, cough, and chest pain. The cough, associated with weight loss, persists. Because of poor performance at football practice, he is advised to see a physician. Lymph node biopsies stained with H and E studies reveal granulomatous inflammation and macrophages engorged with oval structures measuring 2–4 μm. Cultures incubated at room temperature grow powdery white colonies, which on microscopic study have tuberculate spores. The high school student most likely acquired his infection from which of the following?

a. Another human via respiratory secretions
b. Bird excrement
c. Cat feces
d. Contaminated drinking water
e. Desert sand

# Mycology

## Answers

**320. The answer is a.** *(Brooks, pp 649–650, 640–642, 645–646. Levinson, pp 338–341. Murray—2005, pp 791–793, 714–715, 716. Ryan, pp 655–656, 660–664, 670–672.)* Both clinical symptoms and cultural characteristics of the causative agent suggest the diagnosis of this patient as aspergillosis, a common infection seen in immunocompromised hosts. Tuberculosis is unlikely because the patient is tuberculin test negative. The causative fungus for mucormycosis (phycomycosis) produces nonseptate hyphae in culture. *H. capsulatum*, which causes histoplasmosis in humans, grows in yeast form in the infected person. *Candida*, causative agent for candidiasis, does not produce hairy colonies on an agar surface.

**321. The answer is a.** *(Brooks, pp 649–650. Levinson, pp 338–341. Murray—2005, pp 791–793. Ryan, pp 665–667.)* *Aspergillus* species cause infections of the skin, eyes, and ears, and "fungus ball" in the lungs. *Aspergillus* species occur only as molds (not dimorphic). They have septate hyphae that form V-shaped branches, whose walls are parallel. Septate, branching hyphae invading tissue are typically seen in biopsy. On culture, colonies with radiating chains of conidia (photo) are typical. These molds are widely spread in nature, and transmission is by airborne conidia. The organism is very opportunistic in immunocompromised individuals, and antifungal treatment may be difficult.

**322. The answer is e.** *(Brooks, pp 647–649. Levinson, pp 333–337. Murray—2005, pp 788–789. Ryan, pp 674–678, 680–683.)* Thick-walled spores are characteristic of many fungal infections, including blastomycosis, coccidioidomycosis, and histoplasmosis. Observation of these structures in sputum or in tissue should alert the microbiologist to a diagnosis of systemic fungal infection. The presence of encapsulated yeast in clinical specimens may suggest the presence of *Cryptococcus*.

**323. The answer is c.** *(Brooks, pp 629–630. Levinson, pp 331–332. Murray—2005, pp 858–589. Ryan, pp 649–650.)* Hairs infected with both *M. canis* and *M. audouini* fluoresce with a yellow-green color under Wood's light, while

*T. rubrum, T. tonsurans,* and *E. floccosum* do not. But *M. audouini* is an anthropophilic agent of tinea capitis, whereas *M. canis* is zoophilic. *M. canis* is seen primarily in children and is associated with infected cats or dogs.

**324. The answer is b.** *(Brooks, pp 647–649. Levinson, pp 333–337. Murray—2005, pp 788–789. Ryan, pp 669–672.)* Patients with paralysis of their cellular immune system, such as in AIDS, are susceptible to a wide variety of diseases, including infection with *Cryptococcus.* A brain abscess caused by *C. neoformans* is not unusual in patients with AIDS. Initial laboratory suspicion is usually aroused by the presence of encapsulated yeast in the CSF. There also could be other microorganisms as well as noninfectious artifacts that superficially resemble yeast. While *C. neoformans* can be readily cultured, a rapid diagnosis can be made by detecting cryptococcal capsular polysaccharide in CSF or blood. Care must be taken to strictly control the test because rheumatoid factor may cross-react. Once the yeast is isolated, then specific stains as well as panels of assimilatory carbohydrates are available to definitively identify this organism as *C. neoformans.* The patient may also be infected with *P. carinii,* but not in the central nervous system. *P. carinii* has recently been reclassified as a fungus.

**325. The answer is c.** *(Brooks, pp 647–649. Levinson, pp 333–337. Murray—2005, pp 788–789. Ryan, pp 669–672.)* *C. neoformans* occurs widely in nature, particularly in soil contaminated with bird droppings. Human infection occurs when inhalation of the organism occurs. Lung infection is often asymptomatic but can result in pneumonia. Meningitis occurs through dissemination, particularly in immunosuppressed patients. India ink preparations of CSF reveal a budding yeast with a wide, unstained capsule in infected persons.

**326. The answer is e.** *(Brooks, pp 635–636. Levinson, pp 331–332. Murray—2005, pp 759–760.)* Eumycotic mycetoma is a slowly progressing disease of the subcutaneous tissues that is caused by a variety of fungi. The term *Madura foot* has been used to describe the foot lesion. Although several fungi have been isolated in the United States from persons who have mycetoma, *Pseudallescheria boydii* appears to be one of the most common. Other foot infections that may resemble Madura foot are actinomycotic (bacterial) in nature. These are caused by *Nocardia brasiliensis* and *Actinomadura.*

**327. The answer is a.** (*Brooks, pp 642–644. Levinson, pp 333–337. Murray—2005, pp 765–769. Ryan, pp 672–683.*) The key diagnostic finding is the morphology of the yeast isolated from the granulomatous, supurative lesions of the lung. *Blastomyces dermatitidis*, which causes blastomycosis, grows in the yeast form in infected tissues. The bud of growing yeast is attached to the parent cell by a broad base. Although the fungi that cause all other diseases listed in the question grow in yeast form in infected tissues, most buds are attached to the parent cell by a narrow base.

**328. The answer is e.** (*Brooks, pp 632–634. Levinson, pp 331–332. Murray—2005, p 757. Ryan, pp 654–656.*) Cutaneous sporotrichosis, caused by *S. schenckii,* begins at the site of inoculation, usually on an extremity or the face. The organism often is found on thorns of rosebushes. Ulceration is common, and new lesions appear along paths of lymphatic channels. Extracutaneous sporotrichosis is seen primarily in bones and joints. There is no evidence to suggest that any portal of entry besides skin is important.

**329. The answer is b.** (*Brooks, pp 628–629. Levinson, pp 331–332. Murray—2005, pp 748–751.*) The dermatophytes (see figure presented in the question) are a group of fungi that infect only superficial keratinized tissue (skin, hair, nails). They form hyphae and arthroconidia on the skin; in culture, they develop colonies and conidia. Tinea pedis, or athlete's foot, is the most common dermatophytosis. Several topical antifungal agents, such as undecylenic acid, salicylic acid, and ammoniated mercury, may be useful in treatment. For serious infection, systemic use of griseofulvin is effective.

**330. The answer is e.** (*Brooks, pp 645–647. Levinson, pp 338–341. Murray—2005, pp 781–786. Ryan, pp 660–664.*) C. albicans is the most important species of *Candida* and causes thrush, vaginitis, skin and nail infections, and other infections. It is part of the normal flora of skin, mouth, GI tract, and vagina. It appears in tissues as an oval budding yeast or elongated pseudohyphae. It grows well on laboratory media and is identified by germ-tube formation. A vaccine is not available, and serologic and skin tests have little value.

**331. The answer is b.** (*Brooks, pp 645–647. Levinson, pp 338–341. Murray—2005, pp 781–786. Ryan, pp 660–664.*) C. albicans is part of the normal flora of the gastrointestinal tract, mouth, and genital surfaces. Notwithstanding, *C. albicans* causes severe disease, particularly in those patients with compromised immunity. It is generally thought that when *C. albicans* is unable to adhere to mucosa it is nonpathogenic and that production of germ tubes or hyphae plays a major role in colonization and infection of the mucosal epithelial cells by allowing direct penetration of these cells with specific hydrolytic enzymes. While other mutations such as temperature intolerance, metabolic alterations, and structural substitutions may affect the ability of *Candida* to survive, these changes would not affect adherence.

**332. The answer is a.** (*Brooks, pp 649–650. Levinson, pp 333–341. Murray—2005, pp 791–793. Ryan, pp 665–667.*) While all fungi such as *Candida* and *Cryptococcus* are potentially serious in a bone marrow transplant unit (BMTU), the most frequent cause of fungal infection and death is *Aspergillus.* Aspergilli are ubiquitous in the environment. There are instances of multiple infections in new units that have not been monitored prior to opening or in units adjacent to construction projects. Strict precautions should be taken to exclude dust and debris from the BMTU area during construction, but in any event the environment should be monitored for airborne microorganisms, especially *Aspergillus,* prior to opening the unit.

**333. The answer is b.** (*Brooks, pp 640–642. Levinson, pp 333–337. Murray—2005, pp 714–715. Ryan, pp 672–676.*) *H. capsulatum* is a dimorphic fungus that forms two types of spores: tuberculate macroconidia and microconidia. Inhalation of the microconidia transmits infection. Inhaled spores (microconidia) are engulfed by macrophages and develop into yeast forms. Most infections remain asymptomatic; small granulomatous foci heal by calcification. However, pneumonia can occur. The heterophile antibody test is useful for early diagnosis of infectious mononucleosis.

**334. The answer is d.** (*Brooks, p 650. Levinson, pp 338–341. Ryan, pp 678–680.*) This description is a typical picture of mucormycosis occurring in a diabetic patient. The organism is a member of *Phycomycetes,* which forms uniseptate hyphae. In candidiasis, septate hyphae and budding yeast are seen in infected tissues. Nocardiosis, erysipelas, and gas gangrene are not mycotic infections. They are caused by bacteria (*N. asteroides, Streptococcus pyogenes, and Clostridium perfringens* respectively).

**335. The answer is c.** (*Brooks, pp 645–647. Levinson, pp 338–341. Murray—2005, pp 779–787. Ryan, pp 678–680.*) *C. albicans* and *C. tropicalis* are opportunistic fungi, and as part of the normal flora are not transmitted by inhalation. *C. immitis* is a dimorphic fungus, and inhalation of the spores transmits the infection. *Sporothrix* is also a dimorphic fungus, but its portal of entry is cutaneous. *Trychophyton* is a dermatophyte and one of the causes of athlete's foot.

**336. The answer is a.** *(Brooks, pp 649–650. Levinson, pp 338–341. Murray— 2005, pp 717–718, 791–793. Ryan, pp 665–667.)* *Aspergillus* is an opportunistic pathogen that can invade wounds, burns, abraded skin, the cornea, and the outer ear. However, in immunocompromised patients, infection of the wound site is not common. *Aspergillus* does not cause urinary tract infection. In immunocompromised persons, invasive disease occurs. Blood vessel invasion can result in thrombosis and infarction. In pulmonary cavities (due to tuberculosis), "fungus ball" formation can occur, which can be seen on x-ray. Infection of the bronchi can result in allergic bronchopulmonary aspergillosis, characterized by asthmatic symptoms. Thrush is caused by *C. albicans*. Rashes are not usually seen with *Aspergillus* infection.

**337. The answer is b.** *(Brooks, pp 637–639. Levinson, pp 333–337. Murray— 2005, pp 712–714. Ryan, pp 680–683.)* In patients with coccidioidomycosis, a positive skin test to coccidioidin appears 2–21 days after the appearance of disease symptoms and may persist for 20 years without reexposure to the fungus. A decrease in intensity of the skin response often occurs in clinically healthy people who move away from endemic areas. A negative skin test frequently is associated with disseminated disease. CF immunoglobulin G (IgG) antibodies, which may not appear at all in mild disease, rise to a high titer in disseminated disease, a poor prognostic sign. For this reason, a persistent or rising CF titer combined with clinical symptoms indicates present or imminent dissemination. Rarely is the CF titer negative. Most persons infected with *C. immitis* are immune to reinfection.

**338–341. The answers are 338-d, 339-c, 340-b, 341-a.** *(Brooks, pp 623–629. Levinson, pp 331, 338–341. Murray—2005, p 817. Ryan, pp 660–668.)* Fungi that cause opportunistic infections are diverse, and most of them are represented in this group of questions. Infection occurs primarily in the compromised host with underlying diseases such as lymphoma, leukemia, and diabetes. Unfortunately, most of the opportunistic fungi that cause infection are commonly seen in the laboratory as contaminants.

Candidiasis is the most frequent opportunistic infection. While *C. albicans* is most commonly isolated, other species such as *C. tropicalis* and *Torulopsis glabrata* are also seen. The yeasts may be identified biochemically, but *C. albicans* is distinctive in that it produces germ tubes and chlamydospores.

Aspergillosis, caused by a number of species of *Aspergillus*, is characterized in direct smear by septate hyphae, dichotomously branched. *Aspergillus flavus* and *A. fumigatus* are often seen as saprophytes in the laboratory but also account for the major species isolated from patients with aspergillosis. Differentiation of species, as with the zygomycetes, is dependent upon isolation of the fungus and precise morphological examination.

Zygomycosis, a term referring to infection by members of the class Zygomycetes, is caused primarily by *Rhizopus, Mucor,* and *Absidia*. Other zygomycetes such as *Basidiobolus* and *Cunninghamella* are rarely encountered. The lack of septate hyphae on a direct smear may be the initial hint of zygomycosis. However, not uncommonly, the occasional hypha of *Mucor* will have a septum. The genera cannot be differentiated on a direct patient specimen. The organism must be isolated and slide cultures performed to observe the characteristic morphology of these filamentous fungi.

*Rhizopus* species have sporangia that arise from a stolon, while *Mucor* species do not. *Mucor* species have collarettes; *Rhizopus* species do not.

**342. The answer is e.** *(Brooks, pp 650–651. Levinson, pp 78, 344, 354. Murray—2005, pp 798–800. Ryan, pp 685–689.)* *P. carinii* causes pneumonia in immunocompromised patients. Once considered a protozoan, it is not classified as a fungus. Effective chemoprophylactic regimens have resulted in a dramatic decrease in pneumonia deaths in AIDS patients. *P. carinii* has the morphologically distinct forms (trophozoite and cyst) described in the question. Cysts stain well with silver stain. In clinical specimens, trophozoites and cysts are present in a tight mass. *P. carinii* cannot be cultured. The organism is widespread in nature and does not cause disease without immunosuppression. It may represent a member of normal flora.

**343. The answer is e.** *(Brooks, pp 628–632. Levinson, pp 331–332. Murray—2005, pp 748–751. Ryan, p 653.)* Of the available answer choices, only tinea corporis dermatophyte infection will show numerous, smooth-walled macroconidia, with microconidia being absent. *Epidermophyton* species would be a common cause of this kind of rash. Jock itch (tinia cruruis—groin) can involve particularly bad lesions if inappropriate use of topical steroids is involved. This is also called tinea incognito. Tinea or ringworm designations were used because of the dermatophyte infections. Treatment usually consists of thorough removal of infected and dead epithelial structure and application of a topical antifungal medication.

**344. The answer is d.** *(Brooks, pp 632–634. Levinson, pp 331–332. Murray— 2005, p 757. Ryan, pp 654–656.)* *S. schenkii* is a dimorphic fungus that lives on vegetation. A mold with branching septate hyphae and conidia at ambient temperature, it grows as a small budding yeast at 37°C. Following traumatic introduction into the skin, a chronic granulomatous infection occurs with secondary spread to local lymph nodes. For systemic treatment, Amphoteracin B is given. *Malassezia* and *Microsporum* produce superficial infections. *Coccidioides* would be transmitted by airborne mechanisms. *S. chartarum* is the toxic house mold that is so prevalent in current news reports.

**345–349. The answers are 345-b, 346-a, 347-c, 348-c, 349-a.** *(Brooks, pp 216–218, 220, 640–642, 7. Levinson, pp 164, 481s–482s, 333–337. Murray— 2005, pp 417–418, 289–292, 714–715. Ryan, pp 649–650, 676–683.)*

**345. The answer is b.** Actinomycosis is a chronic suppurative and granulomatous infection that produces pyogenic lesions with interconnecting sinus tracts that contain granules composed of microcolonies of bacteria embedded in tissue components. The etiologic agents are closely related to normal oral flora with most cases being due to *Actinomyces israelii*, a facultative anaerobe. The three most common forms are cervicofacial, thoracic, and abdominal, with trauma being the mechanism that introduces these organisms into the mucosa tissues. The bacteria bridge the mucosal surfaces of the mouth, respiratory tract, and lower GI tract. Infection is associated with dental caries, gingivitis, surgical complication, or trauma, as mentioned above. Aspiration may lead to pulmonary infection. Cervicofacial disease presents as a swollen, erythematous process in the jaw area, producing draining fistulas. *A. bovis* seldom causes human disease. Nocardia infection is usually caused by inhalation of the organism and relate to pulmonary infections. *H. capsulatum* could be identified by microscopic examination of exudate, showing large, spherical thick-walled macroconidia with peripheral projections of cell wall materials.

**346. The answer is a.** Sensitivity, in medical diagnosis, is the probability of the test finding disease among those who have the disease or the proportion of people with disease who have a positive test result. Sensitvitiy = true positives/(true positives + false negatives). Specificity is the probability of the test finding NO disease among those who do NOT have the disease or the proportion of people free of a disease who have a negative test. Specificity = true negatives/(true negatives + false positives). Positive Predictive Value (PPV) is the percentage of people with a positive test result who actually have the disease. Negative Predictive Value (NPV) would be the percentage of people who do NOT have the disease. When a diagnostic test or sign has a high sensitivity, a Negative result rules out the diagnosis. When a diagnostic sign or test has a high specificity, a Positive result rules in the diagnosis. In our test question, 25% prevalence (total number of cases of a disease in a given population at a given time) is relatively high. Incidence, for comparison, is the number of cases (especially new cases) in a given population over a period of time. In our example, in order to maximize the chances of finding the true number of disease cases, we would wantthe highest degree of specificity (98%).

**347. The answer is c.** (*Brooks, pp 640–642. Murray—2005, pp 714–715.*) In *H. capsulatum* infection, conidia develop into yeast cells which are engulfed by alveolar macrophages. These may give rise to inflammatory reactions that become granulomatous. In culture at 25°C, *H. capsulatum* develops hyphae with microconidia and large, spherical macroconidia with peripheral projections of cell-wall materials. The macrocondia are also called tuberculate macroconidia. Arthroconidia (arthrospores) result from the fragmentation of hyphal cells of *C. immitis*. Spherules result when arthroconidia are inhaled and enlarge into larger bodies that contain endospores. Spherules can be produced in the laboratory using a complex medium. Sclerotic bodies are found in chromoblastomycosis infections. The fungi reside in soil and vegetation and cause skin infections. In tissue, the fungi appear as spherical brown cells termed muniform or sclerotic bodies that divide by transverse separation. Separation in different planes may give rise to a cluster of 4–8 cells.

**348. The answer is c.** (*Brooks, pp 645–647. Murray—2005, pp 779–787.*) It has long been recognized that fungi may be part of the normal (usual) microbial flora of humans, but their numbers are kept quite low by the competition for food, and the like, by the faster growing bacteria. If some mechanism (broad-spectrum antibiotics) alter the usual flora, these fungi, especially *Candida,* may become efficient opportunists and cause a disease situation. Removal of the antibiotic will allow reestablishment of normal bacterial flora and control *Candida* numbers again.

**349. The answer is a.** (*Brooks, pp 637–639. Murray—2005, pp 712–714.*) Valley fever is caused by *C. immitis.* It is grown on Sabouraud's agar, and the infection is endemic in the semiarid regions of the southwestern United States, as well as Central and South America. Hyphae form chains of arthroconidia (arthrospores) which often develop in alternate cells of a hypha. Individual arthroconidia are released from chains, become airborne and are resistant to harsh environmental conditions. Following inhalation, arthroconidia become spherical, enlarge forming spherules that contain endospores. Such spherules have a thick, refractive cell wall and are diagnostic of *C. immitis.* Blastospores represent conidial formation through a budding process, as seen in yeast or chains of *Cladosporium.* Chlamydospores are large, thick-walled spherical conidia produced from terminal hyphal cells (*C. albicans*). Sporangiospores are sexual structures characteristic of zygomycetes (mitotic spores produced within an enclosed sporangium, of ten supported by one sporangiophore (*Rhizopus, Mucor*).

**350–353. The answers are 350-d, 351-a, 352-d, 353-c.** (*Brooks, pp 628–632. Levinson, pp 331–332. Murray—2005, pp 748–751. Ryan, pp 649–650, 654.*) Dermatomycoses are cutaneous mycoses caused by three genera of fungi: *Microsporum, Trichophyton,* and *Epidermophyton.* These infections are called *tinea* or *ringworm,* a misnomer that has persisted from the days when they were thought to be caused by worms or lice. Tinea capitis (ringworm of the scalp) is due to an infection with *M. canis* or *T. tonsurans.* It usually occurs during childhood and heals spontaneously at puberty. Circular areas on the scalp, with broken or no hair, are characteristic of this disorder. Tinea corporis (ringworm of the body) is caused by *M. canis* and *Trichophyton mentagrophytes.* This disorder affects smooth skin and produces circular pruritic areas of redness and scaling. Both tinea cruris (ringworm of the groin, "jock itch") and tinea pedis (ringworm of the feet, athlete's foot) are caused by *T. rubrum, T. mentagrophytes,* or *E. floccosum.* These common conditions are pruritic and can cause scaling. Tinea versicolor (pityriasis versicolor) is not a dermatomycotic condition but, rather, a superficial mycosis now thought to be caused by M. furfur. The disorder is characterized by chronic but asymptomatic scaling on the trunk, arms, or other parts of the body.

**354. The answer is b.** (Brooks, pp 645–647. Levinson, pp 331–341. Murray— 2005, pp 716, 781–784. Ryan, pp 660–664.) Candida species are normal flora of the skin, mucous membranes, and gastrointestinal tract. The risk of endogenous infection is ever present. Candidiasis is the most common systemic mycosis. Oral thrush develops in most patients with AIDS. Other risk factors include antibiotic use and cellular immunodeficiency. Mucor and Rhizopus are primarily dermatophytes, while Aspergillus is usually derived from an environmental source. While Aspergillus is a significant opportunist, the numbers of cases are much lower than those observed to be caused by Candida. Cryptococcus is usually acquired by inhalation.

**355–356. The answers are 355-c, 356-e.** (Brooks, pp 645–647. Levinson, pp 331–332, 338–341. Murray—2005, pp 716, 781–784.) Candidiasis, cryptococcosis, zygomycosis, and aspergillosis are among the most common opportunistic fungal infections. These fungi are commonly observed in the environment and are innocuous to people with intact host defenses. However, when host defenses are compromised by immunosuppression (AIDS), cytotoxic drugs, diabetes, or devices that breach the normal host defenses, these usually harmless fungi become potent pathogenic microorganisms.

C. albicans is a member of the normal human microflora. This yeast causes such relatively mild infections as "jock itch" and diaper rash. Suppression of cellular immunity often results in more serious yeast infections. Oral candidiasis is one of the earliest and most frequent of the opportunistic infections in patients with AIDS. Diagnosis of invasive candidiasis is difficult, especially when patients are symptomatic and Candida is not recovered from blood specimens. Candidal antibody tests, antigen detection, and metabolite detection have not been successful in differentiating between invasive disease and colonization. The figure presented in Question 338 illustrates C. albicans from a skin smear.

Zygomycosis (sometimes called mucormycosis) is caused by a variety of fungi called zygomycetes. These fungi include Conidiobolus, Rhizopus, and Basidiobolus, which can be differentiated mycologically, but all are characterized by large (6–25 mm), irregularly branched, usually nonseptate hyphae. The differentiation of these fungi clinically is a function of the location of the lesion: limbs and trunk, nose, or brain. *Basidiobolus* lesions are most commonly seen on the arms and legs. *Conidiobolus* is usually found in the nasal mucosa and nasal sinuses. *Rhizopus* infection may start in the nasal tissue but spreads rapidly to the eyes and brain.

**357. The answer is b.** *(Brooks, pp 637–639. Levinson, pp 333–337. Murray—2005, pp 712–714. Ryan, pp 678–683.)* Endemic areas for *C. immitis* are semi-arid regions, particularly the central valleys of California and southern Arizona. The infection rate is highest during the dry months of summer and autumn, when dust is prevalent. Inhalation of arthroconidia can lead to an asymptomatic infection in 60% of individuals. The other 40% may develop a self-limited influenza-like illness. Individuals with cell-mediated immunosuppression may lead to dissemination of endospores by the blood. The most frequent sites involved are skin, bones and joints, and the meninges. Histoplasmosis is usually associated with the central river valleys of the United States, while blastomycocis is endemic primarily in the eastern United States. *M. marinum* is usually associated with fish and water, while *Mycoplasma pneumoniae* transmission is from person to person.

**358. The answer is e.** *(Brooks, pp 632–634. Levinson, pp 331–332, 495s. Murray—2005, p 757. Ryan, pp 654–656.)* *Sporothrix* is a dimorphic fungus that lives on vegetation. While a mold form at ambient temperatures and producing septate hyphae and conidia, the infection almost always follows traumatic introduction into the skin. A chronic granulomatus infection is typical, with local lymph nodes being involved. Multiple lesions (abscesses) may occur along the lymphatics. *Histoplasma, Coccidioides, Cryptococcus,* and *Aspergillus* are usually acquired by inhalation.

**359. The answer is b.** *(Brooks, pp 640–642. Levinson, pp 333–337. Murray—2005, pp 772–775. Ryan, pp 672–676.)* *H. capsulatum* infection is highest in the United States, especially in the Ohio and Mississippi river valleys. Numerous outbreaks have resulted from exposure of many persons to inocula of conidia. These occur when the organism is disturbed from its natural habitat, soil mixed with bird feces or bat guano. Feces provides an excellent culture for fungal growth to occur. Some 80–90% of residents in certain endemic areas may have positive skin tests. Histoplasmosis is not transmissible from person to person.

# Parasitology

## Questions

**DIRECTIONS:** Each question below contains four or more suggested responses. Select the **one best** response to each question.

**360.** Babesiosis, as observed in the figure below, is a tick-borne disease resulting in a febrile illness. Infection with *Babesia* is most commonly observed in which of the following?

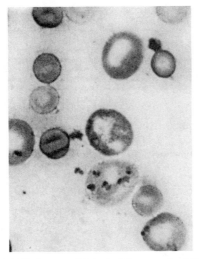

Small ring forms of the WA-1 strain of *Babesia*. (Giemsa stain; 1000× magnification.) *(Reproduced, with permission, from Wilson WR, Sande MA. Current Diagnosis and Treatment in Infectious Disease. New York: McGraw-Hill, 2001: 805.)*

a. AIDS patients
b. Foresters
c. Patients without a spleen
d. Transfusion recipients
e. Transplant recipients

**361.** An AIDS patient presents to his primary care physician with a 2-week history of watery, nonbloody diarrhea. This stool reveals the organism seen in the figure below. Which of the following is the most likely diagnosis?

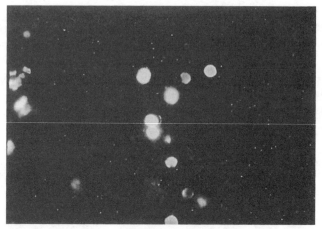

*(Reproduced, with permission, from Wilson WR, Sande MA. Current Diagnosis and Treatment in Infectious Disease. New York: McGraw-Hill, 2001: 827.)*

a. Acid-fast bacilli
b. *Enterocytozoon*
c. *Cryptosporidium*
d. *Cyclospora*
e. Yeast

**362.** A healthy 30-year-old woman consumed half a box of imported raspberries 10 days ago. She experienced a self-limited but prolonged, relapsing watery diarrhea, along with fatigue and low-grade fever. Stool examination revealed oocysts with autofluorescent inclusions and were acid fast. Which of the following is the most likely cause of her infection?

a. *Escherichia coli* 0157:H7
b. *Cyclospora*
c. *Cryptosporidium*
d. *Isospora*
e. *Vibrio*

**363.** In order to exert control over the primary cause of toxoplasmosis of pregnancy, which of the following steps of the life cycle of *Toxoplasma* would be most practical to interrupt?

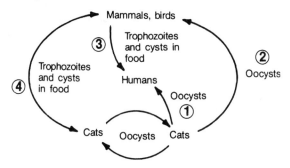

a. Step 1
b. Step 2
c. Step 3
d. Step 4
e. Steps 3 and 4

**364.** A 30-year-old female stored her contact lenses in tap water. She noticed deterioration of vision and visited an ophthalmologist, who diagnosed her with severe retinitis. Culture of the water as well as vitreous fluid would most likely reveal which of the following?

a. *Acanthamoeba*
b. *Babesia*
c. *Entamoeba coli*
d. *Naegleria*
e. *Pneumocystis*

**365.** The diagnostic characteristics of *Plasmodium falciparum* (see figure) are best described by which one of the following statements?

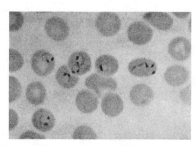

Sequestration of *P falciparum*-infected RBCs in the maternal sinuses of the placenta. This photomicrograph was taken after quinidine therapy. The corresponding peripheral blood smear was almost devoid of parasites. (Hematoxylin and eosin stain; 600× magnification.) *(Reproduced, with permission, from Wilson WR, Sande MA. Current Diagnosis and Treatment of Infectious Diseases. New York: McGraw-Hill, 2001: 798.)*

a. An important diagnostic feature is the irregular appearance of the edges of the infected red blood cell
b. A period of 72 hours is required for the development of the mature schizont, which resembles a rosette with only 8–10 oval merozoites
c. Except in infections with very high parasitemia, only ring forms of early trophozoites and the gametocytes are seen in the peripheral blood
d. Schüffner stippling is routinely seen in red blood cells that harbor parasites
e. The signet-ring-shaped trophozoite is irregular in shape with ameboid extensions of the cytoplasm

**366.** The life cycle of this parasite consists of two stages: the cyst and the trophozoite, as shown in the figure below. Which of the following is the most likely identification of this organism?

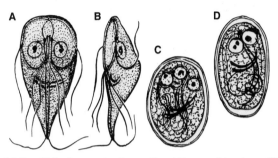

A: "Face" and B: "profile" of vegetative forms; C and D: cysts (binucleate [D] and quadrinucleate stages). 2000×. *(Reproduced, with permission, from Brooks GF et al. Jawetz's Medical Microbiology, 23e. New York: McGraw-Hill, 2004:662.)*

a. *Clonorchis*
b. *Entamoeba*
c. *Giardia*
d. *Pneumocystis*
e. *Trichomonas*

**367.** A divorced working mother takes her 4-year-old child to a day-care center. She has noticed that the child's frequent stools are nonbloody with mucus and are foul smelling. The child has no fever, but does complain of "tummy hurting." The increase of fat in the stool directs the pediatrician's concern toward a diagnosis of malabsorption syndrome associated with which of the following?

a. Amebiasis
b. Ascariasis
c. Balantidiasis
d. Enterobiasis
e. Giardiasis

**368.** A family from a rural area of Central America migrated to the United States. Several members of the family present to a physician with headache, vertigo, and vomiting. Calcified cysts are observed in computed tomography scans, indicating possible cysticercosis. Which of the following statements best describes the basis for the patients' infection and symptoms?

a. Acute intestinal stoppage is less common in beef tapeworm infection
b. Beef tapeworm eggs cause less irritation of the mucosa of the digestive tract
c. Larval invasion does not occur in beef tapeworm infection
d. The adult beef tapeworms are smaller
e. Toxic by-products are not given off by the adult beef tapeworm

**369.** A man coughed up a long (4–6 cm) white worm, and his chief complaint is abdominal tenderness. He reports that he goes to sushi bars at least once a week. The following parasites have been observed in people who eat raw fish: *Anisakis, Pseudoterranova, Eustrongylides,* and *Angiostrongylus.* Which of the following would best differentiate the specific parasitic agent?

a. Antigen detection in tissues
b. Characteristic signs and symptoms
c. Identification of specific species of fish involved
d. Specific antibody tests
e. Study of distinctive morphology of the parasite

**370.** A survey of 100 healthy adults reveals that 80% have IgG antibodies to *Toxoplasma.* Which of the following statements helps to explain this finding?

a. A variety of parasitic infections induce the formation of *Toxoplasma* antibody
b. The IgM test is more reliable than the IgG test for determination of past infections; retesting for IgM would show that most people do not have *Toxoplasma* antibody
c. The potential for *Toxoplasma* infection is widespread, and the disease is mild and self-limiting
d. The test for *Toxoplasma* antibodies is highly nonspecific
e. Toxoplasmosis is caused by eating meat; therefore, all meat eaters have had toxoplasmosis

**371.** A 32-year-old gay man presents to his physician with non-bloody, foul-smelling, greasy stools 3 weeks after travel to Mexico. While certain enteric protozoan and helminthic infections have been long related to contaminated food or water, sexual transmission of these diseases has produced a "hyperendemic" infection rate among gay males. Which of the following organisms is the most likely etiologic cause of this patient's diarrhea?

a. Amebiasis
b. Ascariasis
c. Enterobiasis
d. Giardiasis
e. Trichuriasis

**372.** Analysis of a patient's stool reveals small structures resembling rice grains; microscopic examination shows these to be proglottids. Which of the following is the most likely organism in this patient's stool?

a. *Ascaris lumbricoides*
b. *Enterobius vermicularis*
c. *Necator americanus*
d. *Taenia saginata*
e. *Trichuris trichiura*

**373.** An AIDS patient complains of headaches and disorientation. A clinical diagnosis of *Toxoplasma encephalitis* is made, and *Toxoplasma* cysts are observed in a brain section (see figure below). Which of the following antibody results would be most likely in this patient?

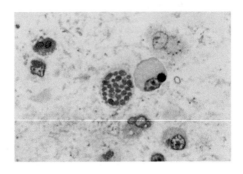

a. IgM nonreactive, IgG nonreactive
b. IgM nonreactive, IgG reactive (low titer)
c. IgM reactive (low titer), IgG reactive (high titer)
d. IgM reactive (high titer), IgG reactive (high titer)
e. IgM reactive (high titer), IgG nonreactive

**374.** A young boy from an impoverished area in Argentina presented to a public health clinic with Romana's sign and a chagoma lesion. Several reduviid insects from the home were shown to the health care workers. In the chronic stage of this disease, where are the main lesions usually observed?

a. Digestive tract and respiratory tract
b. Heart and digestive tract
c. Heart and liver
d. Liver and spleen
e. Spleen and pancreas

**375.** A woman who recently returned from Africa complains of having paroxysmal attacks of chills, fever, and sweating. These attacks last a day or two at a time and recur every 36–48 hours. Examination of a stained blood specimen reveals ringlike and crescent-like forms within red blood cells. Which of the following is the most likely infecting organism?

a. *P. falciparum*
b. *Plasmodium vivax*
c. *Schistosoma mansoni*
d. *Trypanosoma gambiense*
e. *Wuchereria bancrofti*

## Item 376–377

A young man, recently returned to the United States from Vietnam, has severe liver disease. Symptoms include jaundice, anemia, and weakness.

**376.** Which of the following is the most likely etiologic agent, shown in the photomicrographs below?

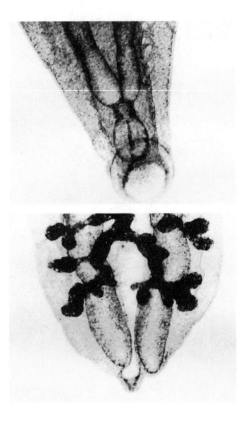

a. *Clonorchis sinensis*
b. *Diphyllobothrium latum*
c. *P. falciparum*
d. *T. saginata*
e. *T. solium*

**377.** An intermediate form of the organism shown in the above photomicrographs lives in which of the following organisms?

a. Cows
b. Mosquitoes
c. Pigs
d. Snails
e. Ticks

**378.** A woman who recently traveled through Central Africa now complains of severe chills and fever, abdominal tenderness, and darkening urine. Her febrile periods last for 28 hours and recur regularly. Which of the following blood smears would most likely be associated with the symptoms described?

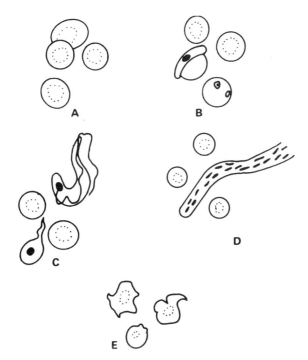

a. A
b. B
c. C
d. D
e. E

**379.** One of the most clinically significant infections in patients with AIDS is *Pneumocystis carinii* pneumonia (PCP). PCP is a treatable disease; therefore, rapid diagnosis is essential. Which of the following is the method of choice for detection of *P. carinii* in respiratory specimens?

a.  Culture in rat lung cells
b.  Direct fluorescent antibody (DFA) microscopy
c.  Indirect fluorescent antibody (IFA) microscopy
d.  Methenamine-silver stain
e.  Toluidine blue stain

**380.** Which of the following protozoa is known only in the trophozoite stage?

a.  *Balantidium coli*
b.  *Entamoeba histolytica*
c.  *Giardia lamblia*
d.  *Toxoplasma gondii*
e.  *Trichomonas vaginalis*

**381.** An international photographer returns to the United States from a global picture assignment. He is seen by his physician, giving his major complaint as diarrhea. Which of the following can be ruled out?

a.  *Echinococcus granulosus*
b.  *Dientamoeba fragilis*
c.  *D. latum*
d.  *G. lamblia*
e.  *Leishmania donovani*

**382.** A "parasite" that most clearly resembles a fungus when examined by molecular techniques, is the initial clinical manifestation in up to 60–90% of patients with AIDS and is considered the gold standard in diagnosis for these individuals. Which of the following is this organism?

a.  *Blastocystis*
b.  *Blastomyces*
c.  *Cryptosporidium*
d.  *Microsporidium*
e.  *Pneumocystis*

**383.** A medical technologist visited Scandinavia and consumed raw fish daily for 2 weeks. Six months after her return home, she had a routine physical and was found to be anemic. Her vitamin $B_{12}$ levels were below normal. Which of the following is the most likely cause of her vitamin $B_{12}$ deficiency anemia?

a. Cysticercosis
b. Excessive consumption of ice-cold vodka
c. Infection with the fish tapeworm *D. latum*
d. Infection with Parvovirus B19
e. Infection with *Yersinia*

**384.** A renal transplant patient is admitted for graft rejection and pneumonia. A routine evaluation of his stool shows rhabditiform larvae. Subsequent follow-up reveals similar worms in his sputum. He has no eosinophils in his peripheral circulation. Which of the following is the most likely organism?

a. *Ascaris*
b. *Hymenolepis*
c. *Loa loa*
d. *Necator*
e. *Strongyloides*

**385.** A 56-year-old male immigrant from Bolivia complains of abdominal pain and cramping. He comments that 2 months previous to his current problems, he had numerous bloody stools every day. Physical findings include right upper quadrant pain over the liver with hepatomegaly. A liver biopsy is performed. Which of the following parasites would most likely be identified in the liver biopsy?

a. *Acanthamoeba*
b. *Ascaris*
c. *Balantidium*
d. *Entamoeba*
e. *Taenia*

**386.** Malaria is a significant worldwide public health problem. The life cycle of *Plasmodium* can be seen in the figure below. Which of the following control methods for malaria is currently effective?

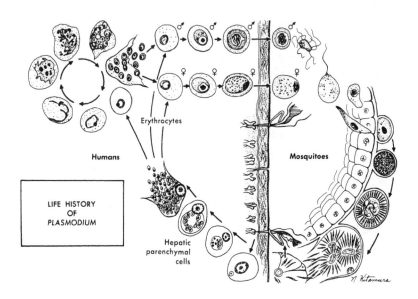

a. Antibiotics
b. A vaccine
c. Chemoprophylaxis
d. Tick repellents
e. White clothing

**387.** Genetically induced changes in the glycoprotein coat of which of the following organisms enhances its escape from the host's immune antibody response?

a. *Trichinella spiralis*
b. *Trichmonas vaginalis*
c. *T. gondii*
d. *T. gambiense*
e. *L. donovani*

**388.** Amebas that are parasitic in humans are found in the oral cavity and the intestinal tract. Which of the following statements best describes these intestinal amebas?

a.  Infection with *E. histolytica* is limited to the intestinal tract
b.  They are usually nonpathogenic
c.  They are usually transmitted as trophozoites
d.  They can cause peritonitis and liver abscesses
e.  They occur most abundantly in the duodenum

**389.** *Schistosoma haematobium* produces a disease characterized by granulomatous reactions to the ova or to products of the parasite at the place of oviposition. Clinical manifestations include which of the following?

a.  Arthropathies
b.  Bladder wall hyperplasia
c.  Cardiac abnormalities
d.  Pulmonary embolism
e.  Hemorrhagic cystitis

**390.** *Borrelia burgdorferi*, the causative agent of Lyme disease, has been isolated from a variety of ticks such as *Ixodes scapularis, Amblyomma, Dermacentor,* and *Ixodes pacificus*. Which of the following statements is true of Lyme disease?

a.  *Dermacentor* and *Amblyomma* are significant vectors of *B. burgdorferi* to humans
b.  Dogs and cats are naturally immune to Lyme disease
c.  *I. scapularis* and *Ixodes dammini* are different types of ticks
d.  Only a small percentage of people who get bitten by a tick develop Lyme disease
e.  White-tailed deer, an important reservoir for *I. scapularis*, are dying because of Lyme disease

**391.** Which of the following infections requires a mosquito for transmission to humans?

a.  Babesiosis
b.  Bancroftian filariasis
c.  Dog tapeworm
d.  Guinea worm
e.  Leishmaniasis

**392.** Which of the following organisms penetrates skin, is endemic in Africa and Latin America, and has a large lateral spine on its eggs?

a.  Clonorchis
b.  Paragonimus
c.  S. haematobium
d.  Schistosoma japonicum
e.  S. mansoni

**393.** Which of the following organisms may be ingested with raw fish, affects the liver, and has an operculated egg?

a.  Clonorchis
b.  Paragonimus
c.  S. haematobium
d.  S. japonicum
e.  S. mansoni

**394.** Which of the following organisms penetrates skin, is endemic in Asia, and has a small lateral spine on its eggs?

a.  Clonorchis
b.  Paragonimus
c.  S. haematobium
d.  S. japonicum
e.  S. mansoni

**395.** Which of the following organisms penetrates skin, is endemic in Africa and the Middle East, has large terminal spines on its eggs, and is found in urine samples?

a.  Clonorchis
b.  Paragonimus
c.  S. haematobium
d.  S. japonicum
e.  S. mansoni

**396.** G. lamblia is best diagnosed by which of the following?

a.  Baermann technique
b.  Dilution followed by egg count
c.  Enzyme immunoassay (EIA)
d.  Examination of a cellophane tape swab
e.  Sigmoidoscopy and aspiration of mucosal lesions

**397.** *E. histolytica* infection is best diagnosed by which of the following?

a.  Baermann technique
b.  Dilution followed by egg count
c.  Enzyme immunoassay (EIA)
d.  Examination of a cellophane tape swab
e.  Sigmoidoscopy and aspiration of mucosal lesions

**398.** The best method for the detection of *Strongyloides* larvae is which of the following?

a.  Baermann technique
b.  Dilution followed by egg count
c.  Enzyme immunoassay (EIA)
d.  Examination of a cellophane tape swab
e.  Sigmoidoscopy and aspiration of mucosal lesions

**399.** *Ascaris* is best observed in human specimens by which one of the following?

a.  Baermann technique
b.  Dilution followed by egg count
c.  Enzyme immunoassay (EIA)
d.  Examination of a cellophane tape swab
e.  Sigmoidoscopy and aspiration of mucosal lesions

**400.** A butcher who is fond of eating raw hamburger develops chorioretinitis. A Sabin-Feldman dye test is positive. This patient is most likely infected with which of the following?

a.  Giardiasis
b.  Schistosomiasis
c.  Toxoplasmosis
d.  Trichinosis
e.  Visceral larva migrans

**401.** A fur trapper complains of sore muscles, has swollen eyes, and reports eating bear meat on a regular basis. He is most at risk for which of the following?

a.  Giardiasis
b.  Schistosomiasis
c.  Toxoplasmosis
d.  Trichinosis
e.  Visceral larva migrans

**402.** A newspaper correspondent has diarrhea for 2 weeks following a trip to St. Petersburg (Leningrad). She is most likely to have which one of the following?

a. Giardiasis
b. Schistosomiasis
c. Toxoplasmosis
d. Trichinosis
e. Visceral larva migrans

**403.** A retired Air Force colonel has had abdominal pain for 2 years; he makes yearly freshwater fishing trips to Puerto Rico and often wades with bare feet into streams. Which of the following should be included in the differential diagnosis?

a. Giardiasis
b. Schistosomiasis
c. Toxoplasmosis
d. Trichinosis
e. Visceral larva migrans

**404.** A teenager who works in a dog kennel after school has had a skin rash, eosinophilia, and an enlarged liver and spleen for 2 years. Which of the following is the most likely cause of this infection?

a. Giardiasis
b. Schistosomiasis
c. Toxoplasmosis
d. Trichinosis
e. Visceral larva migrans

**405.** A protozoan with characteristic jerky motility is most commonly observed in which of the following?

a. Biopsied muscle
b. Blood
c. Duodenal contents
d. Sputum
e. Vaginal secretions

**406.** A helminth that is naturally transmitted by ingestion of pork, bear, or walrus meat could be detected in which of the following?

a. Biopsied muscle
b. Blood
c. Duodenal contents
d. Sputum
e. Vaginal secretions

**407.** A tissue-dwelling trematode that may be found in feces can also be detected in which of the following?

a. Biopsied muscle
b. Blood
c. Duodenal contents
d. Sputum
e. Vaginal secretions

**408.** Cysts of a protozoan adhere to a piece of nylon yarn coiled in a gelatin capsule, which is swallowed. These cysts are usually found in which of the following?

a. Biopsied muscle
b. Blood
c. Duodenal contents
d. Sputum
e. Vaginal secretions

**409.** A parasite resembling malaria that infects both animals and humans and is carried by the same tick that transmits *B. burgdorferi* (the bacterium that causes Lyme disease) would most likely be observed in which of the following?

a. Biopsied muscle
b. Blood
c. Duodenal contents
d. Sputum
e. Vaginal secretions

# Parasitology

## Answers

**360. The answer is c.** *(Brooks, pp 682–683. Levinson, pp 334, 359–360, 501s. Murray—2005, pp 866–867.)* *Babesia* is a tick-borne organism transmitted by *I. scapularis*, the same tick that transmits Lyme disease. *Babesia* is often mistaken for *Plasmodia* (causative organism of malaria) on a blood smear. Patients become anemic and develop hepatosplenomegaly, but patients who are asplenic are at a much greater risk. Transfusion recipients, foresters, and immunosuppressed patients may be at risk of acquiring disease but not to the same extent as those patients who have been splenectomized.

**361. The answer is c.** *(Brooks, pp 684–685. Levinson, pp 345–348. Murray—2005, pp 855–856. Ryan, p 702.)* The figure presented in the question shows a *Cryptosporidium* oocyst stained with a fluorescent-labeled specific antibody. *Cryptosporidium* may also be stained with a modified acid-fast stain but are not acid-fast bacilli. They are smaller than *Cyclospora*, which are yeast size, but larger than *Enterocytozoon*, one of the microsporidia.

**362. The answer is b.** *(Brooks, p 683. Levinson, p 344. Murray—2005, pp 856–858.)* Cyclosporiasis is a newly recognized food- and water-borne infectious disease associated with eating contaminated berries imported from some Central American countries. *Cyclospora* are moderately acid-fast but twice the size of *Cryptosporidium*. Patients usually have frequent diarrhea for up to 3 weeks and usually suffer only malaise and fatigue. The disease is self-limiting, but relapses can occur. *Isospora* infection in the United States occurs primarily in patients with AIDS. *Isospora* cysts also autofluoresce and stain acid fast but are at least twice the size of *Cyclospora* oocysts.

**363. The answer is a.** *(Brooks, pp 685–687. Levinson, pp 353–354. Murray—2005, p 882. Ryan, pp 722–727.)* *T. gondii* may be acquired by inhalation of oocysts in cat feces. It is difficult to control the habits of cats unless they are housed and not let out. Pregnant human females should avoid changing cat litter boxes. While ingestion of oocysts in raw meat may also lead to toxoplasmosis, inhalation of oocysts is the primary cause, particularly among pregnant women in the United States.

**364. The answer is a.** (*Brooks, pp 676–677. Levinson, pp 344, 359–360. Murray—2005, pp 869–870. Ryan, p 733.*) *Acanthamoeba* is a free-living ameba, as is *Naegleria*. *Naegleria* usually causes severe, often fatal, meningoencephalitis, while *Acanthamoeba* is uncommonly isolated from contact lens fluid and patients with retinitis who do not store their lenses under sterile conditions. Acanthamoeba can be grown on nonnutrient agar plates using *E. coli* as a food source. They are identified microscopically with use of a nonspecific fluorescent stain.

**365. The answer is c.** (*Brooks, pp 677–682. Levinson, pp 349–353. Murray— 2005, pp 864–867. Ryan, p 712.*) *P. falciparum* infection is distinguished by the appearance of ring forms of early trophozoites and gametocytes, both of which can be found in the peripheral blood. The size of the RBC is usually normal. Double dots in the rings are common.

**366. The answer is c.** (*Brooks, pp 662–663. Levinson, pp 366–367. Murray— 2005, pp 850–852. Ryan, pp 745–748.*) *Giardia* exists in both trophozoite and cyst form. The "trophs" are fragile and not commonly seen in stools. The cysts are infectious. *Giardia* is the most common parasitic disease in the United States. It is commonly contracted from drinking cyst-contaminated water. Chlorine does not kill *Giardia* cysts, but contaminated water can be made cyst-free by filtration.

**367. The answer is e.** (*Brooks, pp 662–663. Levinson, pp 366–367. Murray— 2005, pp 850–852. Ryan, pp 745–748.*) *G. lamblia* is the only common protozoan found in the duodenum and jejunum. Trophozoites are commonly found in the duodenum and do not penetrate the tissues. Four nuclei cysts (infective stage) can remain viable for up to 4 months. Excystation is via digestive enzymes. The mechanical irritation to tissues leads to diarrhea, with increased fat and mucus in the foul-smelling stool. Malabsorption syndrome (vitamin A and fats) leads to weight loss, anorexia, electrolyte imbalance, and abdominal cramps. Children and immunocompromised individuals are most significantly affected. Giardiasis should be considered in the differential diagnosis of any "traveler's diarrhea."

**368. The answer is c.** (*Brooks, pp 688–691, 696. Levinson, pp 361–364. Murray—2005, pp 907–910. Ryan, pp 793–797.*) Both beef tapeworm (*T. saginata*) and pork tapeworm (*T. solium*) can, in the adult form, cause disturbances of intestinal function. Intestinal disorder is due not only to direct irritation but also to the action of metabolic toxic wastes. In addition, *T. saginata*, because of its large size, may produce acute intestinal blockage. Unlike *T. saginata*, *T. solium* produces cysticercosis, which results in serious lesions in humans (in *T. saginata*, the cysticercus—encysted larvae stage—develops only in cattle).

**369. The answer is e.** (*Brooks, pp 689t, 691t. Levinson, p 342.*) The consumption of raw fish products in Asian restaurants, especially the growing popularity of sushi and sashimi, has led to a variety of infections, most of which are characterized by symptoms consistent with intestinal blockage or meningitis. The parasites are tissue nematodes and parasites of marine mammals. Fish, squid, and other edible marine life are often secondary hosts. The most reliable way to differentiate the specific helminth is by examination of the whole worm or by histologic examination of the parasites in tissue sections.

**370. The answer is c.** (*Brooks, pp 685–687. Levinson, pp 353–354, 499s. Murray—2005, p 882. Ryan, pp 722–727.*) Serologic tests, such as the Sabin-Feldman dye test and indirect immunofluorescence, have shown that a high percentage of the world's population has been infected with *T. gondii*. In adults, clinical toxoplasmosis usually presents as a benign syndrome resembling infectious mononucleosis. However, fetal infections are often severe and associated with hydrocephalus, chorioretinitis, convulsions, and death. Acute toxoplasmosis is best diagnosed by an IgM capture assay. In most patients, specific IgM antibody disappears within 3–6 months.

**371. The answer is d.** (*Brooks, pp 662–663. Levinson, pp 366–367. Murray—2005, pp 850–852. Ryan, pp 745–748.*) The infection rate with *G. lamblia* in male homosexuals has been reported to be from 21–40%. These high prevalence rates are probably related to three factors: the endemic rate, the sexual behavior that facilitates transmission (the usual barriers to spread have been interrupted), and the frequency of exposure to an infected person.

**372. The answer is d.** (*Brooks, pp 687–693. Levinson, pp 372–382. Murray—2005, pp 879–881. Ryan, pp 793–795.*) *Enterobius* (pinworm), *Ascaris* (roundworm), *Necator* (hookworm), and *Trichuris* (whipworm) are roundworms, or nematodes. *T. saginata* (tapeworm), a segmented flatworm, affects the small intestine of humans. Tapeworm segments, called *proglottids,* appear in the stool of infected persons.

**373. The answer is b.** *(Brooks, pp 685–687, 759t. Levinson, pp 319, 353–354, 499s. Murray—2005, p 882. Ryan, pp 722–727.)* One of the leading causes of death among AIDS patients is central nervous system toxoplasmosis. It is thought that *Toxoplasma* infection is a result of reactivation of old or preexisting toxoplasmosis. Occasionally, the infection may be acquired by needle sharing. Because the disease is a reactivation of old or preexisting toxoplasmosis, routine quantitative tests for IgM antibody are usually negative, and IgG titers are low ($\leq$1:256, IFA). More sophisticated methods, such as IgM capture or IgG avidity, may reveal an acute response.

**374. The answer is b.** *(Brooks, pp 665, 668–671. Levinson, pp 344–345. Murray—2005, pp 875–876. Ryan, pp 695, 757–760.)* American trypanosomiasis (Chagas' disease) is produced by *T. cruzi,* which is transmitted to humans by the bite of an infected reduviid bug. After multiplication, the tissues most likely to be affected in the chronic stage of the disease are the cardiac muscle fibers and the digestive tract. A diffuse interstitial fibrosis of the myocardium results and may lead to heart failure and death. The inflammatory lesions in the digestive tract that are seen in the esophagus and colon produce considerable dilatation. Chagas' disease has not been an important disease in the United States; most cases have been imported, although there are a few reports of endogenous disease in the southern United States.

**375. The answer is a.** *(Brooks, pp 677–682. Levinson, pp 349–353. Murray—2005, pp 861–865. Ryan, p 712.)* The febrile paroxysms of *Plasmodium malariae* malaria occur at 72-hour intervals; those of *P. falciparum* and *P. vivax* malaria occur every 48 hours. The paroxysms usually last 8–12 hours with *P. vivax* malaria but can last 16–36 hours with *P. falciparum* disease. In *P. vivax, Plasmodium ovale,* and *P. malariae* infections, all stages of development of the organisms can be seen in the peripheral blood; in malignant tertian (*P. falciparum*) infections, only early ring stages and gametocytes are usually found.

**376. The answer is a.** *(Brooks, pp 688–690t. Levinson, pp 370–371. Murray—2005, pp 898–900. Ryan, pp 807–808.)* The Chinese liver fluke, *C. sinensis,* is a parasite of humans that is found in Japan, China, Korea, Taiwan, and Indochina. Humans usually are infected by eating uncooked fish. The worms invade bile ducts and produce destruction of liver parenchyma. Anemia, jaundice, weakness, weight loss, and tachycardia may follow. Treatment is likely to be ineffectual in heavy infections, but chloroquine can destroy some of the worms.

**377. The answer is d.** *(Brooks, pp 688–690t. Levinson, pp 367–371. Murray— 2005, pp 898–900. Ryan, pp 807–808.)* The life cycle of *C. sinensis* is similar to that of other trematodes. A mollusk is characteristically the first intermediate host of trematodes. For *C. sinensis,* snails perform this role.

**378. The answer is b.** *(Brooks, pp 677–682. Levinson, pp 349–353. Murray— 2005, pp 861–865. Ryan, pp 711–722.)* The case history presented in the question is characteristic of infection with *P. falciparum,* the causative agent of malignant tertian malaria. The long duration of the febrile stage rules out other forms of malaria. The presence of ringlike young trophozoites and crescent-like mature gametocytes—as represented in the illustration below— as well as the absence of schizonts is diagnostic of *P. falciparum* malaria.

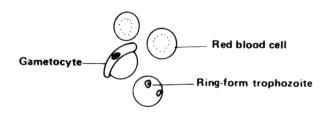

**379. The answer is b.** *(Brooks, pp 650–651. Levinson, p 341. Murray— 2005, pp 798–800. Ryan, pp 685–689.)* Both methenamine-silver and toluidine blue stain pneumocysts nonspecifically. These preparations are difficult to read because background material may nonspecifically stain black or blue. *P. carinii* cannot be routinely cultured from human specimens. Both IFA and DFA tests are FDA-approved and available for detection of *P. carinii.* The advantage of DFA is that it is quicker (45–60 minutes versus 3 hours), and there is less nonspecific fluorescence observed in the preparation. Recent evidence suggests that *Pneumocystis* is a fungus. Polymerase chain reaction (PCR), in sputum especially, increases sensitivity but reduces specificity.

**380. The answer is e.** *(Brooks, pp 663–665. Levinson, pp 344, 348–349s. Murray—2005, pp 582–583. Ryan, pp 742–745.)* *T. vaginalis* is the only protozoan listed where the trophozoite is the diagnostic and infective stage that feeds on the mucosal surface of the vagina (bacteria and leukocytes). The troph possesses a short, undulating membrane (one-half of the body) and four anterior flagella. No cyst stage exists. A persistent vaginitis with a frothy and foul-smelling discharge with burning, itching, and increased frequency of urination is common. Three to six million women in the United States are infected annually, while males are usually asymptomatic. Wet mounts examined in the laboratory reveal trophozoites with rapid, jerky, and nondirectional motion.

**381. The answer is a.** *(Brooks, pp 688t, 697. Levinson, pp 362, 365–366. Murray—2005, pp 912–913. Ryan, pp 799–801.)* *E. granulosis* causes hydatid disease. The definitive hosts are dogs. Sheep, cattle, and humans are intermediate hosts. The adult tapeworm does not occur in humans. In the herbivores (infected by grazing where eggs have been deposited by carnivore feces), the eggs hatch and release hexacanths. These penetrate the gut and pass to other tissues (liver, viscera, muscle, and brain). Humans are only infected from dog feces and develop hydatid cysts, as described for herbivores. Diarrhea, therefore, does not occur with *E. granulosis* human infections, whereas the other four choices can routinely present with diarrhea.

**382. The answer is e.** *(Brooks, pp 650–651. Levinson, p 341. Murray—2005, pp 798–800. Ryan, pp 685–689.)* One of the multiple criteria for classification of AIDS is the development of PCP. *Pneumocystis* is a fungus formerly thought to be a parasite that was classified with the sporozoa. PCP may also be seen in patients with congenital or other acquired cellular immune dysfunction. Most patients with AIDS are given prophylactic aerosolized pentamidine or TMP-SMX for PCP. PCP is easily diagnosed in respiratory secretions by a DFA test. Both the microsporidia and *Cryptosporidium* are intestinal parasites that also infect patients with AIDS, but these microorganisms cause protracted diarrhea. Both *Blastocystis* and *Blastomyces* are yeasts and should not be confused with *Pneumocystis* or each other.

**383. The answer is c.** *(Brooks, pp 697–698. Levinson, pp 362, 365–366. Murray—2005, pp 910–911. Ryan, pp 797–798.)* Consumption of raw fish causes endemic diphyllobothriasis in Scandinavia and the Baltic countries. While most people do not become ill, a small percentage (2%) develops vitamin $B_{12}$ deficiency anemia. The adult fish tapeworm has an affinity for vitamin $B_{12}$ and may induce a serious megaloblastic anemia. Parvovirus B19 causes acute hemolytic anemia primarily in immunosuppressed patients. *Yersinia* infection is common in Scandinavia but is not fish-borne and does not cause anemia. The larval stage of *T. solium* is called *cysticercus*. Humans usually acquire cysticercosis by ingestion of food and water contaminated by infected human feces.

**384. The answer is e.** (*Brooks, pp 693–694. Levinson, pp 375, 378. Murray—2005, pp 885–887. Ryan, pp 763, 774–777.*) Strongyloidiasis may be observed in three phases: cutaneous, pulmonary, and intestinal. The pulmonary presentation of *Strongyloides* in patients with AIDS is the most common. Often, all body fluids will contain larvae. Prognosis is poor. *Necator* must be distinguished from *Strongyloides* by microscopy. Gross appearances are similar.

**385. The answer is d.** (*Brooks, pp 671–674. Levinson, pp 343–346, 498s. Murray, pp 847–849.*) *E. histolytica* is a pathogenic species that is capable of causing disease, such as colitis or liver abscess, in humans. *E. dispar* is indistinguishable from *E. histolytica* by usual laboratory tests but only exists in humans as an asymptomatic carrier state and does not cause colitis. Infection with *E. histolytica* is prevalent in Central and South America, southern and western Africa, the Far East, and India. Poor sanitation and lower socioeconomic conditions favor the spread of the disease. In the United States, those who travel to endemic areas, homosexual males, and institutionalized persons are at increased risk of infection. *Acanthamoeba* species are free-living amebas in soil and water and usually cause infections of the skin, encephalitis, and kerititis. Ascaris is a nematode and is transmitted by ingestion. They hatch in the small intestine, and larvae migrate to the pulmonary alveoli. From here, they induce a cough and are swollowed by the host, maturing in the small intestine. *B. coli* is a ciliate, infecting the lining of the large intestine, cecum, and terminal ilium. *Taenia* species (beef and pork) are ingested in undercooked meat. Only *T. solium* (pork) may occasionally involve liver if cystericercosis occurs.

**386. The answer is c.** (*Brooks, pp 681–682. Levinson, pp 349–353. Murray—2005, pp 861–867. Ryan, pp 711–722.*) Prophylaxis for malaria should be considered whenever a person is traveling in a malaria-endemic area. Drugs consist of mefloquine or chloroquine and Fansidar. Other control measures such as draining swamps, protective clothing and netting, and insect repellents are also effective. There is no currently available vaccine for malaria.

**387. The answer is d.** *(Brooks, pp 668–671. Murray—2005, pp 872–876. Ryan, p 902.)* African trypanosomiasis (sleeping sickness) is caused by *T. brucei gambiense* and *T. brucei rhodensiense* and transmitted by tsetse flies. From the fly's salivary glands, the trypomastigotes enter the host's blood and lymph and eventually the CNS. The trypomastigotes reproduce by binary fission and are infective for biting tsetse flies. During the course of trypanosome infection, the number of parasites in the blood and lymph tissues fluctuates according to the host's immune response. An increase in parasite number is related to the proliferation of parasite subpopulations that express an antigenically new or variant glycoprotein coat. Each parasite carries genes encoding multiple, variant surface glycoproteins (VSG) with only one VSG being expressed at any one time. These changes lead to evasion of the immune system and produce challenges for vaccine development. The other parasites listed do not exhibit this ability to change surface glycoproteins.

**388. The answer is d.** *(Brooks, pp 671–674. Levinson, pp 343–346, 498s. Murray—2005, pp 847–849. Ryan, pp 733–738.)* Of the intestinal amebas, *Entamoeba hartmanni, E. coli, Entamoeba polecki,* and *Entamoeba nana* are considered nonpathogenic. *E. histolytica* is distinctively characterized by its pathogenic potential for humans, although infection with this protozoan is commonly asymptomatic (causing "healthy carriers"). Symptomatic amebiasis and dysentery occur when the trophozoites invade the intestinal wall and produce ulceration and diarrhea. Peritonitis can occur, with the liver the most common site of extraintestinal disease. The life cycle of the *ameba* is simple by comparison. There is encystment of the troph, followed by excystation in the ileocecal region. The trophs multiply and become established in the cecum, where encystation takes place and results in abundant amebas, cysts, and trophozoites. Infection is spread by the cysts, which can remain for weeks or months in appropriately moist surroundings.

**389. The answer is e.** *(Brooks, pp 661, 695t. Levinson, pp 367–370. Murray— 2005, pp 902–905. Ryan, pp 803, 808–813.)* Although the chronic stage of

proliferation within tissues is distinctive in the different forms of schistosomiasis, a granulomatous reaction to the eggs and chemical products of the
schistosome occurs in all forms of the disease. *S. haematobium* commonly
involves the distal bowel and the bladder, as well as the prostate gland and
seminal vesicles. Bladder calcification and cancer may ensue. S. haemotobium
infection has the flukes located in the vesicular plexis, and granulomatous
formations occur in the bladder and ureters. Hematuria is a common complaint. With prolonged infection, fibrosis, ureteral obstruction, and chronic
renal failure may occur. *S. mansoni* affects the large bowel and the liver;
presinusoidal portal hypertension, splenomegaly, and esophageal varices
may be complications. Pulmonary hypertension, often fatal, may be seen
with *S. mansoni* and *S. japonicum* disease. Eggs may be found in an
unstained specimen of rectal mucosa or in stool. Urine microscopy and
liver biopsy, when warranted, often prove positive. Schistosomiasis is best
prevented by the elimination of the parasite in snails before human infection occurs.

**390. The answer is d.** *(Brooks, pp 336–338. Levinson, pp 24, 32, 169–172.
Murray—2005, pp 433–436. Ryan, pp 434–437.)* In the United States,
*B. burgdorferi*, the causative agent of Lyme disease, has two principal vectors: *I. scapularis* in the eastern and midwestern United States and *I. pacificus* in the western United States. The ticks are tiny and can easily be
missed. Fortunately, relatively few people who are bitten by ticks develop
Lyme disease. Lyme disease, usually with joint involvement, is also seen in
veterinary patients such as dogs, cats, and horses. White-tailed deer and
small rodents are an important reservoir for these ticks. *B. burgdorferi* has
been isolated from mosquitoes and *Dermacentor* and *Amblyomma* ticks as
well as from several *Ixodes* species. However, the isolation of the bacterium
from these ticks is not sufficient evidence to indicate that they transmit the
disease to humans.

**391. The answer is b.** *(Brooks, pp 689–694. Levinson, pp 373–374,
379–380. Murray—2005, pp 888–890. Ryan, pp 695–779, 784–785.)* W. ban-
*crofti* is the cause of bancroftian filariasis or filarial elephantiasis. Control of
the mosquito vectors (culex, anopheles, and Aedes) is the most significant
mechanism to control human infections. A disease of the tropics and sub-
tropics, adults live in the lymphatics of a host and cause lymph blockage of
the feet, arms, genitals, and breasts. Enlargement of the affected body part

(elephantiasis) can then occur. Babesiosis is caused by tick-borne *Babesia microti.* Leishmaniasis is spread by a sand fly (Phlebotomus) vector. Guinea worms (*Dracunculus medinensis*) has an aquatic life cycle involving copepods (water fleas). Dog tapeworms would routinely be transmitted by fecal contamination.

**392–395. The answers are 392-e, 393-a, 394-d, 395-c.** *(Brooks, pp 694–696. Levinson, pp 367–371. Murray—2005, pp 897–905. Ryan, pp 803, 809–813.)* The life cycle of the medically important trematodes (or flukes) involves a sexual cycle in humans and an asexual cycle in snails. The schistosomes can penetrate the skin, whereas *Clonorchis* and *Paragonimus* are ingested, usually in fish or seafood. These flukes can be easily differentiated morphologically by the appearance of the egg. Schistosome eggs have an identifiable spine, and both *Clonorchis* and *Paragonimus* eggs are operculated; that is, they have what appears to be a cover that opens. Serological tests are not useful. Many patients with schistosomiasis are asymptomatic, but disease may become chronic, resulting in malaise, diarrhea, and hepatosplenomegaly (an enlarged liver and spleen). *Clonorchis* infection usually causes upper abdominal pain but can also cause biliary tract fibrosis. Paragonimiasis is characterized by a cough, often with bloody sputum, and pneumonia. Praziquantel is the treatment of choice for these flukes.

**396–399. The answers are 396-c, 397-e, 398-a, 399-b.** *(Brooks, pp 661–702. Levinson, pp 343–347, 376, 378. Murray—2005, pp 837–846. Ryan, pp 695–696, 733–738, 745–748, 769–771, 774–777.)* It is not uncommon that repeated stool specimens do not reveal the suspected parasite. Also, microscopic analysis of stool may not reveal parasite load when such data are necessary. For these reasons, other techniques are available to identify parasites as well as to quantitate them.

The diagnosis of giardiasis is usually made by detecting trophozoites and cysts of *G. lamblia* in consecutive fecal specimens. Alternatively, a gelatin capsule on a string (enterotest) can be swallowed, passed to the duodenum, and then retrieved after 4 hours. The string is then examined for *Giardia*. A recent innovation is the introduction of an EIA for *G. lamblia*. The EIA is more sensitive than microscopy, can be performed on a single stool specimen, and does not depend on the presence of entire trophozoites and cysts.

During sigmoidoscopy, a curette or suction device may be used to scrape or aspirate material from the mucosal surface. Cotton swabs should not be used. A direct mount of this material should immediately be examined for *E. histolytica* trophozoites, and then a permanent stain made for subsequent examination.

The Baermann technique may be helpful in recovering *Strongyloides* larvae. Essentially, fecal material is placed on damp gauze on the top of a glass funnel that is three-quarters filled with water. The larvae migrate through the damp gauze and into the water. The water may then be centrifuged to concentrate the *Strongyloides*.

Worm burdens may be estimated by a number of microscopic methods. While not often done, such procedures may provide data on the extent of infection or the efficacy of treatment of hookworms, *Ascaris,* or *Trichuris*. Thirty thousand *Trichuris* eggs per gram, 2000–5000 hookworm eggs per gram, and one *Ascaris* egg are clinically significant and suggest a heavy worm burden.

A cellophane tape swab is used to trap pinworms crawling out of the anus during the night. The tape is then examined microscopically for *Enterobius*.

**400–404. The answers are 400-c, 401-d, 402-a, 403-b, 404-e.** (*Brooks, pp 685–687, 688–691, 662–663, 687–690. Levinson, pp 346–347, 353–354, 367–370, 378–379, 381–382. Murray—2005, pp 882–883, 907–910, 850–852, 902–905, 882–883. Ryan, pp 695–696, 723–727, 746–748, 779–784, 809–813.*) All the diseases listed in the question have significant epidemiologic and clinical features. Toxoplasmosis, for example, is generally a mild, self-limiting disease; however, severe fetal disease is possible if pregnant women ingest *Toxoplasma* oocysts. Consumption of uncooked meat may result in either an acute toxoplasmosis or a chronic toxoplasmosis that is associated with serious eye disease. Most adults have antibody titers to *Toxoplasma,* and thus would have a positive Sabin-Feldman dye test.

Trichinosis most often is caused by ingestion of contaminated pork products. However, eating undercooked bear, walrus, raccoon, or possum meat also may cause this disease. Symptoms of trichinosis include muscle soreness and swollen eyes.

Although giardiasis has been classically associated with travel in Russia, especially St. Petersburg (Leningrad), many cases of giardiasis caused by contaminated water have been reported in the United States as well. Diagnosis is made by detecting cysts in the stool. In some cases, diagnosis may be very difficult because of the relatively small number of cysts present. Alternatively, an EIA may be used to detect *Giardia* antigen in fecal samples.

Schistosomiasis is a worldwide public health problem. Control of this disease entails the elimination of the intermediate host snail and removal of streamside vegetation. Abdominal pain is a symptom of schistosomiasis.

Visceral larva migrans is an occupational disease of people who are in close contact with dogs and cats. The disease is caused by the nematodes *Toxocara canis* (dogs) and *Toxocara cati* (cats) and has been recognized in young children who have close contact with pets or who eat dirt. Symptoms include skin rash, eosinophilia, and hepatosplenomegaly.

**405–409. The answers are 405-e, 406-a, 407-d, 408-c, 409-b.** *(Brooks, pp 663–664, 693–694, 690, 696, 662–663, 682–683. Levinson, pp 344, 346–347, 348, 359, 368, 378–379. Murray—2005, pp 852–853, 887–888, 900–902, 848–849, 850–852. Ryan, pp 695–696, 741–745, 746–748, 779, 781–784, 803, 805–807.)* T. vaginalis, an odd-looking protozoan, moves with a jerky, almost darting motion. Trichomoniasis, a bothersome vaginal infection, can be diagnosed by observing this organism in a wet mount of vaginal secretions. It may be washed out in the urine as well. *T. vaginalis* can be grown in special media, and there are now several products available for direct detection of the organism.

*T. spiralis* causes trichinosis, a parasitic disease that is usually mild and results in muscle pain and a mild febrile illness. However, fulminant fatal cases have been described. Humans, who are accidental hosts, become infected by ingesting cysts that are in the muscle of animals. Most infections still come from pork, although regulations on pig feeding have markedly reduced the incidence. Laboratory diagnosis is by serology or demonstration of the larvae in the muscle tissue.

*Paragonimus westermani* is a lung fluke. This trematode infects lung tissue and is seen not only in sputum but also in feces because infected patients swallow respiratory secretions. Paragonimiasis is contracted by ingesting the metacercariae that are encysted in crabs or crayfish.

*Giardia* infection may be difficult to diagnose by stool examination, as patients may shed the cysts intermittently. When symptoms persist and the stool examination is negative, then duodenal contents may be sampled directly with the enterotest. The patient swallows a gelatin capsule that contains a coiled string. The other end is attached to the patient's face. The gelatin capsule dissolves, and *Giardia* organisms, if present, adhere to the string within a 4-hour period. The string is retrieved and examined microscopically. Alternatively, an enzymatic immunoassay can detect *Giardia* antigen directly in a single specimen of feces.

*Babesia* is a sporozoan parasite transmitted by the bite of *I. scapularis*, the same tick that carries *B. burgdorferi*. Reproduction of this parasite occurs in erythrocytes and may resemble *Plasmodium* species when blood smears are examined. *Babesia* is endemic in the northeastern United States, particularly in the islands of Massachusetts. Laboratory diagnosis is made by examining blood smears for this parasite, or by detection of specific antibody. Babesiosis clinically resembles malaria.

# Immunology

## Questions

**DIRECTIONS:** Each question below contains four or more suggested responses. Select the **one best** response to each question.

**Item 410–413**

Hypersensitivity reactions are exaggerated or inappropriate immune responses that can sometimes result in damage to the host instead of providing protection. The four main types are represented below.

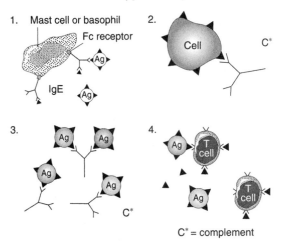

**410.** A 13-year-old male with cystic fibrosis develops repeated episodes of pneumonia resulting in multiple hospitalizations. Previous antibiotic treatment resulted in severe rash, fever, and systemic anaphylaxis almost immediately. A penicilloyl-polylysine skin test yields positive results. Which of the following best illustrates the type of hypersensitivity reaction associated with this clinical scenario?

a. 1
b. 2
c. 3
d. 4

**411.** After playing in the bushes during a camping trip, a 7-year-old girl complains of intense itching and blistering of the hands, arms, and legs. Which of the following is the most likely condition and which is the representative hypersensitivity diagram, respectively, from those presented above?

a. Contact dermatitis and 2
b. Contact dermatitis and 3
c. Contact dermatitis and 4
d. Arthus reaction and 1
e. Arthus reaction and 2
f. Arthus reaction and 3

**412.** Skin testing is useful in the diagnosis of which of the following?

a. 1 and 2
b. 1 and 3
c. 1 and 4
d. 2, 3, and 4

**413.** Rh disease and Goodpasture's syndrome are best represented by which of the following?

a. 1 and 2
b. 2 and 3
c. 2 and 4
d. 2 only
e. 3 only

## Item 414–415

A 7-month-old male infant presented to the emergency department with severe middle ear and upper respiratory tract infections, which responded promptly to antibiotics. Two months later he was again admitted, this time with *Streptococcus pneumoniae* pneumonia. After several more episodes of bacterial infections, genetic testing was done and the presence of a defective B-cell tyrosine kinase gene (*btk* gene or *X-LA* gene) was revealed. In addition, physical examination detected very small tonsils.

**414.** Which of the following is the most likely diagnosis?

a. Ataxia telangiectasia
b. Bruton's agammaglobulinemia
c. Chronic granulomatous disease
d. Late (C5, C6, C7, C8, C9) complement deficiency
e. Thymic aplasia (DiGeorge's syndrome)

**415.** Which of the following pathogens presents the most serious threat to this child?

a. *Chlamydia trachomatis*
b. Measles virus
c. *Mycobacterium tuberculosis*
d. Varicella-zoster virus (VZV)

**Item 416–417**

Flow cytometry of blood from an HIV positive patient yielded a CD4:CD8 ratio < 1.

**416.** This ratio best represents a major decline in which of the following cell types and its associated cell surface proteins?

a. B lymphocytes; MHC I, IgM, B7, CD19, CD20
b. Cytotoxic T lymphocytes; MHC I, TCR, CD3
c. Cytotoxic T lymphocytes; MHC I, TCR, CD3, CD28
d. Helper T lymphocytes; MHC I, TCR, CD3
e. Helper T lymphocytes; MHC I, TCR, CD3, CD28
f. Macrophages; MHC I, MHC II, CD14

**417.** Which of the following best represents the "costimulatory signal" pair that occurs between cellular surface proteins associated with the reduced cell type represented in the CD4:CD8 ratio <1?

a. B7 (B cell) and CD28 (T cell)
b. B7 (B cell) and CD4 (T cell)
c. CD40L (B cell) and CD40 (T cell)
d. MHC Class I (B cell) and CD4 (T cell)
e. MHC Class II (B cell) and CD8 (T cell)

**418.** A young girl has had repeated infections with *Candida albicans* and respiratory viruses since she was 3 months old. As part of the clinical evaluation of her immune status, her responses to routine immunization procedures should be tested. In this evaluation, the use of which of the following vaccines is contraindicated?

a. Bacillus Calmette-Guerin (BCG)
b. *Bordetella pertussis* vaccine
c. Diphtheria toxoid
d. Inactivated polio
e. Tetanus toxoid

**419.** A 7-year-old male developed normally until 7 years of age, then suddenly developed progressive personality and intellect deterioration leading to dementia, and finally death within 1 year of symptoms. His history reveals a severe measles attack at the age of 1. Labs indicate elevated measles antibody levels in both the serum and cerebrospinal fluid (CSF) with no antibody to the M protein. A latent measles-like viral infection and, presumably, a defect in cellular immunity is associated with which of the following diseases?

a. Creutzfeldt-Jakob disease
b. Epstein-Barr virus (EBV) infection
c. Multiple sclerosis (MS)
d. Progressive multifocal leukoencephalopathy (PML)
e. Subacute sclerosing panencephalitis (SSPE)

**420.** A 31-year-old patient suffering from recurrent episodic intestinal hemorrhages from a severe form of Crohn's disease decides to undergo surgery to resect his terminal ileum. The surgeon orders two units of blood to be preserved for possible use during the surgery. The patient decides to store one unit of his own blood and one unit of his 35-year-old brother's blood with the blood bank. This type of donation is most like which of the following transplantation terminology (patient's blood:brother's blood)?

a. allograft:allograft
b. allograft:autograft
c. autograft:allograft
d. autograft:autograft
e. autograft:isograft (syngeneic graft)

**421.** While learning to ride his tricycle, a young boy falls and scrapes his knee. About 3 weeks later he falls again, reinoculating the same wound with the same antigen. The following graph shows the sequential alteration in the type and amount of antibody produced after an immunization. (Inoculation of antigen occurs at two different times, as indicated by the arrows.) Curve A and curve B each represent a distinct type of antibody. The class of immunoglobulin represented by curve B has which of the following characteristics?

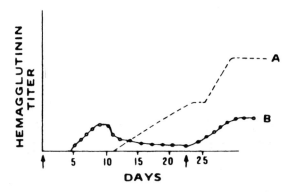

a. A composition of four peptide chains connected by disulfide links
b. A symmetric dipeptide
c. An appearance in neonates at approximately the third month of life
d. An estimated molecular weight of 150,000
e. The human ABO isoagglutinin

**422.** A 27-year-old female presents to the emergency room with a temperature of 103, severe fatigue, weight loss, and joint pain. During the history and physical, the patient reports that she stopped taking her aspirin and corticosteroids to control her condition. A butterfly-type rash over her cheeks, a sensitivity to light, and a heart murmur are apparent. The patient also reports a history of a progressively developing arthritis and glomerulonephritis. Labs further indicate anemia, leukopenia, and thrombocytopenia. This condition is best diagnosed by the presence of which of the following?

a. anticentromere antibodies
b. anti-dsDNA antibodies
c. antimitochondrial antibodies
d. antineutrophil antibodies
e. anti-TSH receptor antibodies

**423.** A 29-year-old highly promiscuous male with a fever, rash, weight loss, general malaise, and a purulent urethral discharge presents to an STD clinic for the first time. Suspecting a gonococcal infection, the physician obtains a specimen and sends it to the lab for an initial enzyme-linked immunosorbent assay (ELISA) test, a widely used method for detecting antigen. The figure below demonstrates an ELISA for detection of antigen. One of the problems with (ELISA) is nonspecific reactivity due to nonspecific antibody present in the reaction. Of the four steps depicted, A, B, C, and D, which one may be the major cause of nonspecificity?

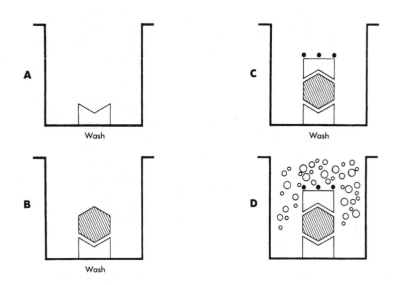

a. A
b. B
c. C
d. D

**424.** An Ouchterlony gel diffusion plate shows the reaction of a polyspecific serum against several antigen preparations. The center well in Figure 1 contains polyspecific antiserum, first bleed; the center well in Figure 2 contains polyspecific antiserum, second bleed; NS is normal saline. In this situation, cross-reaction can be recognized between antigen X and which of the following antigens?

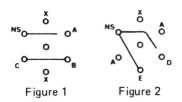

Figure 1        Figure 2

a. A
b. B
c. C
d. D
e. E

**425.** A 1-year-old male patient presents with marked susceptibility to opportunistic infections with bacteria such as *Escherichia coli* and *Staphylococcus aureus* and *Aspergillus*. Examination findings reveal granulomatous abscesses in the lungs, ataxia, nystagmus, and photophobia. Biochemical analysis reveals the deficiency of the central enzyme in the respiratory burst pathway via an inability to reduce nitroblue tetrazolium (NBT) dye. The deficient enzyme and reaction are represented by which of the following?

a. $NADPH + 2O_2 \xrightarrow{\text{NADPH oxidase}} NADP^+ + 2O_2^- + H^+$

b. $2O_2^- + 2H^+ \xrightarrow{\text{Superoxide dismutase}} H_2O_2 + O_2$

c. $H_2O_2 + Cl^- \xrightarrow{\text{Myeloperoxidase}} H_2O + OCl^-$

d. $\tfrac{1}{2}O_2 + \text{arginine} \xrightarrow{\text{NO synthase}} NO + \text{citrulline}$

e. $2H^+ + 2e^- + \tfrac{1}{2}O_2 \xrightarrow{\text{Oxidase}} H_2O$

f. $2H_2O_2 \xrightarrow{\text{Catalase}} 2H_2O + O_2$

**426.** Chromosomal analysis of a patient suffering from a lymphoma revealed the following result:

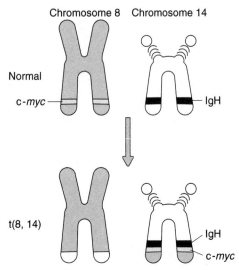

(*Reproduced, with permission, from Parslow TG et al.* Medical Immunology, *10e. New York: McGraw-Hill, 2001, 113.*)

According to the above figure, the patient has which of the following?

a.  Anaplastic large cell lymphoma
b.  Burkitt's lymphoma
c.  Follicular lymphoma
d.  Mantle cell lymphoma

**427.** Which of the following statements best applies to the diagram?

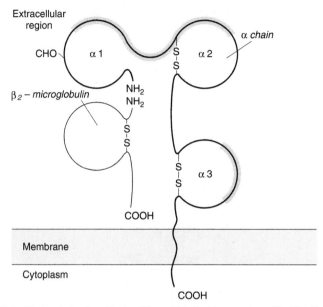

*(Modified, with permission, from Parslow TG et al. Medical Immunology, 10e. New York: McGraw-Hill, 2001, 85.)*

a. Depicts the cell-membrane MHC product associated with narcolepsy
b. Essential for the transplacental passage of antibody
c. Found on memory T and B lymphocytes
d. Present on macrophages but not neutrophils
e. Represents the secretory component associated with IgA
f. Required for recognition of processed antigen by $T_H1$ and $T_H2$ lymphocytes

**428.** A 19-year-old college student develops a rash. She works part-time in a pediatric AIDS clinic. Her blood is drawn and tested for specific antibody to the chickenpox virus (varicella-zoster). Which of the following antibody classes would you expect to find if she is immune to chickenpox?

a. IgG
b. IgA
c. IgM
d. IgD
e. IgE

## Questions 429–431

**429.** A 34-year-old male patient visits a physician with complaints of fatigue, weight loss, night sweats, and "swollen glands." The physician observes that he has an oral yeast infection. Which of the following tests would most likely reveal the cause of the patient's problems?

a. A human T-lymphotropic virus type I (HTLV-I) test
b. A test for *C. albicans*
c. A test for CD8 lymphocytes
d. A test for infectious mononucleosis
e. An HIV ELISA test

**430.** The figure below demonstrates a Western blot for HIV. Based on these results, and assuming a repeatedly reactive ELISA HIV screening test, which of the following is the best course of action?

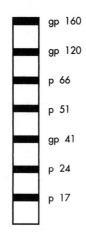

gp 160

gp 120

p 66

p 51

gp 41

p 24

p 17

a. Consider anti-HIV therapy
b. Inform the patient that the test is falsely positive
c. Order an HIV RNA test
d. Repeat the test immediately
e. Wait 6 weeks and repeat the test

**431.** A 30-year-old male patient requests a routine HIV test. The HIV ELISA is weakly positive and is repeated with the same results. The Western blot result is as shown in the preceding figure. The patient denies any risk factors for HIV. Which of the following is the most likely cause of a falsely positive HIV test?

a. A recent flu shot
b. A yeast infection
c. Naturally occurring HIV antibody
d. Test cross-reactivity with Epstein-Barr virus
e. Test cross-reactivity with HTLV

**432.** Patients with C5 through C9 complement deficiencies are most likely to be susceptible to which of the following infections?

a. AIDS
b. Giardiasis
c. Histoplasmosis
d. Neisserial infection
e. Pneumococcal infection

**433.** As part of the management of a 28-year-old male with acute onset of Crohn's disease of the small bowel, you decide to treat him with a new cocktail of mouse-human chimeric antibodies to reduce his intestinal inflammation and cachexia. To which of the following sets of proteins are these antibodies directed?

a. IL-1, IL-2, IL-3
b. IL-2, IL-12, TNF-α
c. IL-2, TGF-β, TNF-α
d. IL-1, IL-6, TNF-α
e. IL-2, IL-3, IL-12

**434.** A mother and newborn are exposed to a pathogen while at the hospital for a routine checkup and breastfeeding clinic. This same pathogen had infected the mother about a year previously, and she had successfully recovered from the subsequent illness. Immunity may be innate or acquired. Which of the following best describes acquired immunity with respect to the newborn?

a. Complement cascade
b. Increase in C-reactive protein (CRP)
c. Inflammatory response
d. Maternal transfer of antibody
e. Presence of natural killer (NK) cells

**435.** A 35-year-old male patient presents with numerous subcutaneous hemorrhages. History and physical exam reveal that he has been taking sedormid (a sedative) for the past week. Laboratory tests indicate normal hemoglobin and white blood cell levels with significant thrombocytopenia (very low platelet count). You suspect that he has developed a drug-induced type II hypersensitivity reaction. This reaction may occur if the drug does which of the following?

a. Activates T cytotoxic cells
b. Acts as a hapten
c. Induces mast cell degranulation releasing mediators such as histamine, leukotrienes, and prostaglandins
d. Induces oxygen radical production through the respiratory burst pathway
e. Persists in macrophages

**436.** After learning of a family history of humoral immunity deficiency during an office visit with a patient 6 months pregnant, a radial immunodiffusion assay is ordered on fetal serum. The test reveals no humoral immunity problems and normal results in all respects. According to this test, the normal level of which fetally-made immunoglobulin is the highest in the fetus?

a. IgA
b. IgD
c. IgE
d. IgG
e. IgM

**437.** Antibodies (immunoglobulins) are extremely important proteins involved in the adaptive immune response whose functions involve the neutralization of toxins and viruses, the opsonization of microbes, and the activation of complement. Which of the following statements is true of immunoglobulins?

a. Digestion of an IgG antibody molecule with papain yields two F(ab) arms, which are unable to agglutinate or precipitate antigen, by cleaving the antibody unit on the C terminus side of the sulfhydryl bridge binding the heavy chain
b. In humans, there are approximately twice as many Ig molecules with κ than λ light chains
c. In the three-dimensional structure of Ig, there is little if any flexibility in the hinge region between the Fc and two F(ab) portions
d. Normally, IgG makes up 20% of the antibody concentration and migrates in the gamma globulin fraction of serum protein separation
e. Pepsin digestion of an IgG molecule cleaves the antibody unit on the N-terminus side of the sulfhydryl bridge binding the heavy chains
f. The two arms of an antibody molecule are different in that they recognize different epitopes

**438.** A 31-year-old male patient complains of fatigue, yeast infection in his mouth, and enlarged lymph nodes under his arms. He says that he was involved in "high-risk" behavior 6 years ago while on a trip to eastern and southern Africa. He also indicates that his "HIV test" was negative. Which of the following options is most appropriate?

a. Initiate treatment for HIV disease
b. Order a test for human T cell leukemia virus (HTLV)
c. Order an HIV-1 RNA PCR
d. Order an HIV test that would include antibodies to HIV-1 and HIV-2
e. Repeat the test for HIV-1

**439.** A laboratory analysis report of a specific fraction of a patient's lymphocytes indicates the following:

HLA, B, and C+, PHA+, CD3−, CD16+, CD11a/CD18+, CD56+, and in vitro blastogenesis with IL-12

What are the lymphocytes this set describes?

a. B lymphocytes
b. Cytotoxic T lymphocytes
c. Natural killer cells
d. T helper 1 subset
e. T helper 2 subset

**440.** The complement system plays a key role in the host defense process. Which of the following components of this system is the most important in chemotaxis?

a. C1q
b. C3a
c. C3b
d. C4a
e. C5a

**441.** A 7-year-old child presents to your clinic during flu season with a severe headache, sinus congestion, fever, sore throat, and cough. Respiratory secretions reveal detectable levels of the cytokine interferon. Which of the following is the mechanism of action of this cytokine?

a. Binds extracellular virus particles and prevents cellular adherence
b. Upregulates the synthesis of secretory proteins that bind and inhibit the virus particles
c. Disrupts viral and cellular protein synthesis, leading to cellular apoptosis
d. Inhibits viral protein synthesis by degrading viral mRNA
e. Downregulates cellular protein synthesis, leading to decreased levels of viral receptors on the cytoplasmic membrane

**442.** Soon after birth a newborn undergoes heart transplantation surgery at a local medical center. Transplantation of tissue and organs is a common procedure whose success depends largely on the "self" vs. "nonself" interactions. Survival of allografts is increased by choosing donors with few major histocompatibility complex (MHC) mismatches with recipients and by use of immunosuppression in recipients. Which of the following procedures is the most useful measure of immunosuppression?

a. Administration of corticosteroids to recipient
b. Administration of immunoglobulin to recipient
c. Destruction of donor B cells
d. Destruction of donor T cells
e. Lymphoid irradiation of donor

**443.** Relative to the primary immunological response, secondary and later booster responses to a given hapten-protein complex can be associated with which one of the following?

a. Antibodies that are less efficient in preventing specific disease
b. Decreased antibody avidity for the original hapten-protein complex
c. Increased antibody affinity for the hapten
d. Lower titers of antibody
e. Maintenance of the same subclass, or idiotype, of antibody produced

**444.** You are managing a 3-year-old female patient with a fever of unknown origin. Her serum is tested for antibodies against *Haemophilus influenzae*. A precipitation test conducted by the clinical laboratory yields the following results:

Serum (Antibody) Dilutions

| Undiluted serum | 1:2 | 1:4 | 1:8 | 1:16 | 1:32 | 1:64 | 1:128 | 1:256 |
|---|---|---|---|---|---|---|---|---|
| − | | + | + | + | + | + | + | − | − |

From this data, which of the following can be concluded?

a. Postzone occurs at undiluted 1:2; zone of equivalence occurs at 1:2–1:64; and prozone occurs at 1:128
b. The negative reactions at 1:128 and 1:126 are false negatives
c. The patient has antibodies against *H. influenzae*, the titer is 64, and the dilution 1:64
d. The patient has antibodies against *H. influenzae*, the dilution is 64, and the titer 1:64
e. The patient does not have antibodies against *H. influenzae* since the reaction is negative with undiluted serum
f. The patient should be immunized against *H. influenzae*
g. The test needs to be repeated because the results cannot be interpreted

**445.** Of the five immunoglobulin classes, IgA is the main immunoglobulin of secretions from the genital, respiratory and intestinal tracts. As a result, IgA antibody is the first line of defense against infections at the mucous membrane. It is usually an early specific antibody. Which of the following statements regarding IgA is true?

a. Complement fixation tests for IgA antibody will be positive if specific IgA antibody is present
b. IgA can be destroyed by bacterial proteases
c. IgA is absent in colostrum
d. IgA is not found in saliva; therefore, an IgA diagnostic test on saliva would have no value
e. IgA is a small molecule with a molecular weight of 30,000 kDa

**446.** A 60-year-old male presents with severe jaudice to the local walk-in clinic. History and physical reveal a 30-year history of alcohol consumption and drug abuse. Blood tests reveal elevated AST and ALT levels and the presence of Hepatitis B and, as a result, reduced complement levels. Complement is a series of important host proteins that provide protection from invasion by foreign microorganisms. Which of the following statements best describes complement?

a. Complement inhibits phagocytosis
b. Complement is activated by IgE antibody classes
c. Complement plays a minor role in the inflammatory response
d. Complement protects the host from pneumococcal infection through C1, C2, and C4
e. Microorganisms agglutinate in the presence of complement but do not lyse

**447.** Radial immunodiffusion and immunoelectrophoresis on a young patient to evaluate his humoral immunity is done. Which of the following immunoglobulin has no known function, is found in the serum in low concentrations, and is present on the surface of B lymphocytes (may function as an antigen receptor)?

a. IgG
b. IgA
c. IgM
d. IgD
e. IgE

**448.** A young patient with severe recurrent pyogenic bacterial infections, but with normal T cell and B cell numbers, arrives at the hospital. Testing reveals that this patient's CD4 T helper cells have a defect in CD40 ligand. As a result, humoral immunity evaluation reveals a significant elevation in the levels of which immunoglobulin, present as a monomer on B cell surfaces, as a pentamer in serum, and is initially seen in the primary immune response?

a. IgG
b. IgA
c. IgM
d. IgD
e. IgE

**449.** A patient with a long history of the consumption of poorly cooked pork meat presents with generalized myalgia and a low-grade fever. Striated muscle biopsy reveals multiple cysts. Eosinophilia is also present with elevated levels of which of the following immunoglobulins most likely involved in parasitic infections?

a. IgG
b. IgA
c. IgM
d. IgD
e. IgE

**450.** A patient with cerebellar problems and spider angiomas is diagnosed with a combined T-cell and B-cell deficiency known as ataxia-telangiectasia. In addition to a defect in this patient's DNA repair enzymes, which immunoglobulin is the primary antibody in saliva, tears, and intestinal and genital secretions, and is also deficient in this illness?

a. IgG
b. IgA
c. IgM
d. IgD
e. IgE

**451.** With four subclasses, which immunoglobulin is the predominant antibody in the secondary immune response and has the greatest concentration of the five immunoglobulin classes in the fetus?

a. IgG
b. IgA
c. IgM
d. IgD
e. IgE

**452.** A 15-year-old boy was bitten by an Ixodes tick while camping with his parents and presents 1 week later with fatigue, fever, headache, and a reddish rash over his trunk and extremities. Positive IgM antibody (1:200) to *Borrelia burgdorferi* is associated with which of the following?

a. Acute Lyme disease
b. Fifth disease
c. Possible hepatitis B infection
d. Possible subacute sclerosing panencephalitis (SSPE)
e. Susceptibility to chickenpox

**453.** A small child presents with a low-grade fever, coryza, sore throat, a bright red rash on his cheeks, and a less intense erythematous rash on his body. Elevated IgG and IgM antibody titers to Parvovirus suggest a diagnosis of which of the following?

a. Acute Lyme disease
b. Fifth disease
c. Possible hepatitis B infection
d. Possible subacute sclerosing panencephalitis (SSPE)
e. Susceptibility to chickenpox

**454.** Blood from a woman at a local pregnancy clinic is analyzed for antibody titers to known pathogens. A negative varicella antibody titer in this young woman signifies which of the following?

a. Acute Lyme disease
b. Fifth disease
c. Possible hepatitis B infection
d. Possible subacute sclerosing panencephalitis (SSPE)
e. Susceptibility to chickenpox

**455.** A patient with severe jaundice and liver failure has an increased antibody titer to delta agent. You should suspect which of the following?

a. Acute Lyme disease
b. Fifth disease
c. Possible hepatitis B infection
d. Possible subacute sclerosing panencephalitis (SSPE)
e. Susceptibility to chickenpox

**456.** A patient with progressively developing neurological disease degeneration has an elevated cerebrospinal fluid (CSF) antibody titer to measles virus. You should suspect which of the following?

a. Acute Lyme disease
b. Fifth disease
c. Possible hepatitis B infection
d. Possible subacute sclerosing panencephalitis (SSPE)
e. Susceptibility to chickenpox

**457.** A 2-year-old patient presents to the pediatrician for a routine visit. History and physical reveal recurrent infections, and enlarged small blood vessels of the skin and conjunctivas. In addition, the physician notices irregular movements most akin to staggering. Suspecting an immune dysfunction, molecular testing reveals a defect in DNA repair enzymes. This autosomal recessive immune deficiency disorder usually is associated with which of the following?

|    | **Humoral** | **Cellular** |
|----|-------------|--------------|
| a. | Normal      | Normal       |
| b. | Normal      | Deficient    |
| c. | Deficient   | Normal       |
| d. | Deficient   | Deficient    |
| e. | Elevated    | Elevated     |

**458.** A 10-month-old male infant with recurrent *Haemophilus influenzae* infections presents to the emergency room with otitis media, sinusitis, and in severe respiratory distress. Immunological testing reveals the absence of B cells and a destructive mutation in the tyrosine kinase gene. This X-linked recessive immune disorder is usually associated with which of the following?

| | **Humoral** | **Cellular** |
|---|---|---|
| a. | Normal | Normal |
| b. | Normal | Deficient |
| c. | Deficient | Normal |
| d. | Deficient | Deficient |
| e. | Elevated | Elevated |

**459.** Amniocentesis conducted during genetic counseling of a pregnant woman reveals a fetal adenosine deaminase deficiency. This autosomal-recessive immunodeficiency is usually associated with which of the following?

| | **Humoral** | **Cellular** |
|---|---|---|
| a. | Normal | Normal |
| b. | Normal | Deficient |
| c. | Deficient | Normal |
| d. | Deficient | Deficient |
| e. | Elevated | Elevated |

**460.** A young child with spastic paralysis presents to the emergency room. Blood tests reveal hypocalcemia. This immune disorder is usually associated with which of the following?

| | **Humoral** | **Cellular** |
|---|---|---|
| a. | Normal | Normal |
| b. | Normal | Deficient |
| c. | Deficient | Normal |
| d. | Deficient | Deficient |
| e. | Elevated | Elevated |

**461.** A 10-month-old patient with recurrent pyogenic infections, eczema, and severe bleeding (thrombocytopenia) is diagnosed with Wiskott-Aldrich syndrome. This immune disorder is usually associated with which of the following?

|     | **Humoral** | **Cellular** |
| --- | --- | --- |
| a. | Normal | Normal |
| b. | Normal | Deficient |
| c. | Deficient | Normal |
| d. | Deficient | Deficient |
| e. | Elevated | Elevated |

**462.** An autograft of a burn victim is best described by which one of the following statements?

a. Transplant from one region of a person to another region
b. Transplant from one person to a genetically identical person
c. Transplant from one species to the same species
d. Transplant from one species to another species

**463.** Transplantation involving tissue from two brothers possessing identical HLA genes is best described by which one of the following statements?

a. Autograft: Transplant from one region of a person to another region
b. Isograft: Transplant from one person to a genetically identical person
c. Allograft: Transplant from one species to the same species
d. Xenograft: Transplant from one species to another species

**464.** A 21-year-old patient in severe kidney failure receives a kidney from his 30-year brother. This type of transpalntation is best described by which of the following statements?

a. Autograft: Transplant from one region of a person to another region
b. Isograft: Transplant from one person to a genetically identical person
c. Allograft: Transplant from one species to the same species
d. Xenograft: Transplant from one species to another species

**465.** During the infancy days of cardiac transplantation, nonhuman primate hearts were transplanted into humans to save lives. This type of transplantation is best described by which one of the following statements?

a. Autograft: Transplant from one region of a person to another region
b. Isograft: Transplant from one person to a genetically identical person
c. Allograft: Transplant from one species to the same species
d. Xenograft: Transplant from one species to another species

**466.** Humoral immunity evaluation mainly consists of measuring the amount of IgG, IgM, and IgA in the patient's serum. These three immunoglobulins represent three distinct isotypes. An isotype is characterized by which of the following statements?

a. Determinant exposed after papain cleavage to an F(ab) fragment
b. Determinant from one clone of cells and probably located close to the antigen-binding site of the immunoglobulin
c. Determinant inherited in a Mendelian fashion and recognized by cross-immunization of individuals in a species
d. Heavy-chain determinant recognized by heterologous antisera
e. Species-specific carbohydrate determinant on the heavy chain

**467.** An allotype is characterized by which of the following statements?

a. Determinant exposed after papain cleavage to an F(ab) fragment
b. Determinant from one clone of cells and probably located close to the antigen-binding site of the immunoglobulin
c. Determinant inherited in a Mendelian fashion and recognized by cross-immunization of individuals in a species
d. Heavy-chain determinant recognized by heterologous antisera
e. Species-specific carbohydrate determinant on the heavy chain

**468.** Antibodies produced from hybridomas are extremely useful clinically for their monoclonal properties. These antibodies have the same idiotype. An idiotype is characterized by which of the following statements?

a. Determinant exposed after papain cleavage to an F(ab')2 fragment
b. Determinant from one clone of cells and probably located close to the antigen-binding site of the immunoglobulin
c. Determinant inherited in a Mendelian fashion and recognized by cross-immunization of individuals in a species
d. Heavy-chain determinant recognized by heterologous antisera
e. Species-specific carbohydrate determinant on the heavy chain

**469.** A 30-year-old male presents to the emergency room with difficulty breathing and abdominal pain. Upon physical exam, you notice diffuse areas of nondependent, nonpitting swelling without pruritus, with predilection for the face, especially the perioral and periorbital areas. You also notice swelling in the mouth, pharynx, and larynx. Laboratory analysis of blood drawn from this patient indicates a complement problem. Which of the following is most likely?

a. High C4, C2, and C3
b. High C1 and normal level of C1 esterase inhibitor
c. High C1 esterase inhibitor and high C4
d. High C1 esterase inhibitor and low C4
e. Low C1 esterase inhibitor and high C4
f. Low C1 esterase inhibitor and low C4
g. Low C4 and high C2

**470.** A 45-year-old businesswoman arrives in your office with vague abdominal complaints. She has noticed melenic stool. Upon performing a sigmoidoscopy, you find a 4-cm mass in the upper colon. You should immediately order a blood test for which of the following tumor markers?

a. Alpha-fetoprotein
b. Antitumor antibody
c. Antitumor light chains
d. Carcinoembryonic antigen
e. Human chorionic gonadotropin
f. Prostate-specific antigen

### Item 471–472

An 18-year-old male heroin addict, who practices the sharing of needles at a "shooting gallery," is positive in the screening test for AIDS.

**471.** This patient is most likely to be immunodeficient because of which one of the following?

a. A genetic defect in chromosome 14
b. A low T helper lymphocyte count
c. An atrophied thymus
d. NADPH enzyme deficiency
e. Insufficient B-cell maturation

**472.** Since a false positive is possible, the physician orders a confirmatory test. Which of the following best describes the standard confirmatory test, and what this test checks for, respectively?

a. Complement fixation test; antibodies against the virus
b. Enzyme-linked immunosorbent assay; antigens of the virus
c. Radioimmunoassay; specific antibodies against the virus
d. Western blot; antigens of the virus
e. Western blot; specific antibodies against the virus

**473.** A pregnant 21-year-old Rh-negative female is about to deliver. The baby's father is determined to be Rh-positive. To reduce the chance for the development of hemolytic disease of the newborn, which of the following procedures should you order?

a. Administration of anti-Rh antibodies to the fetus postdelivery
b. Administration of anti-Rh antibodies to the mother postdelivery
c. Immediate blood transfusion of the suspected father
d. Immediate blood transfusion of the mother with Rh-positive blood
e. Infusion of immune serum globulin into the fetus
f. Intravenous infusion of the Rh antigen into the mother

## Item 474–475

An 8-month-old male infant with a history of chronic diarrhea, otitis media, and several episodes of pneumonia presents to your clinic with gingivostomatitis (due to herpes simplex virus) and oral candidiasis (thrush). You immediately order an x-ray and a blood workup. X-ray and laboratory blood analysis reveal the absence of a thymic shadow and absence of B lymphocytes, respectively. History taken from the infant's mother reveals a rash evident at birth.

**474.** Which of the following diseases is most likely present in this infant?

a. Ataxia-telangiectasia
b. Bruton's agammaglobulinemia
c. Chediak-Higashi syndrome
d. Chronic granulomatous disease
e. Chronic mucocutaneous candidiasis
f. Hereditary angioedema
g. Severe combined immunodeficiency syndrome (SCID)
h. Thymic aplasia (DiGeorge's syndrome)
i. Wiskott-Aldrich syndrome

**475.** Which of the following is the best therapy for this infant?

a. Antifungal agents
b. Blood transfusion
c. Bone marrow transplant
d. IgG from pooled random donors
e. Immunization with attenuated vaccines

**476.** A 5-year-old child arrives at the emergency department minutes after being bitten by a black widow spider. You immediately inject gamma globulin in the form of an antivenom. This type of immunization is referred to as which of the following?

a. Artificial active immunization
b. Artificial passive immunization
c. Natural active immunization
d. Natural passive immunization
e. Adoptive immunization

**477.** A patient with an increased susceptibility to viral, fungal, and protozoa infection would be expected to have a deficiency in which of the following cell types?

a. B lymphocytes
b. Macrophages
c. Natural killer cells
d. Neutrophils
e. T lymphocytes

**Item 478–479**

An 18-year-old female visits her local medical clinic presenting with a now chronic productive cough, general malaise, and fever. Previous visits for this same problem resulted in prescriptions for penicillin and cephalosporins, which proved ineffective. Suspecting *Mycoplasma pneumoniae*, caused by an organism that lacks a cell wall, complement fixation tests are ordered. Complement fixation (CF) testing is an important serological tool. One has to understand the conditions under which complement is bound, and RBCs are lysed.

**478.** Anti-*Mycoplasma* antibody + complement + hemolysin-sensitized red blood cells (RBCs) + anti-RBC antibody results in which of the following?

a. Complement is bound; RBCs are lysed
b. Complement is bound; RBCs are not lysed
c. Complement is not bound; RBCs are lysed
d. Complement is not bound; RBCs are not lysed
e. Complement is not bound; RBCs are agglutinated

**479.** Anti-*Mycoplasma* antibody + *Mycoplasma* antigen + complement + hemolysin-sensitized RBCs + anti-RBC antibody results in which one of the following?

a. Complement is bound; RBCs are lysed
b. Complement is bound; RBCs are not lysed
c. Complement is not bound; RBCs are lysed
d. Complement is not bound; RBCs are not lysed
e. Complement is not bound; RBCs are agglutinated

**480.** While walking through a field, a 28-year-old woman is stung by a bee. Within 10 minutes, she has asthmatic-like symptoms. This type of hypersensitivity reaction can be correctly characterized by which of the following sequences of steps?

a. Allergen, chemical mediators, sensitization, allergen, IgE, symptoms
b. Allergen, IgE, sensitization, allergen, chemical mediators, symptoms
c. Allergen, sensitization, IgE, allergen, chemical mediators, symptoms
d. Sensitization, allergen, chemical mediators, allergen, IgE, symptoms
e. Sensitization, IgE, allergen, symptoms, allergen, chemical mediators

**481.** Finding IgG antibodies to core antigen, antibodies to e antigen, and antibodies to surface antigen reflects which of the following?

a. Acute infection (incubation period)
b. Acute infection (acute phase)
c. Postinfection (acute phase)
d. Immunization
e. HBV carrier state

**482.** Finding HBsAg positive and HBeAg positive reflects which of the following?

a. Acute infection (incubation period)
b. Acute infection (acute phase)
c. Postinfection (acute phase)
d. Immunization
e. HBV carrier state

**483.** Finding HBsAg positive, HBeAg positive, and IgM core antibody positive reflects which of the following?

a. Acute infection (incubation period)
b. Acute infection (acute phase)
c. Postinfection (acute phase)
d. Immunization
e. HBV carrier state

**484.** Finding HBsAg positive, no antibodies to HBsAg, and other tests variable reflects which of the following?

a. Acute infection (incubation period)
b. Acute infection (acute phase)
c. Postinfection (acute phase)
d. Immunization
e. HBV carrier state

**485.** Finding antibodies to HBsAg reflects which of the following?

a. Acute infection (incubation period)
b. Acute infection (acute phase)
c. Postinfection (acute phase)
d. Immunization
e. HBV carrier state

**486.** A 15-year-old male is rushed to the emergency room with a temperature of 103 degrees Farenheit, severe headache, and stiff neck. Upon physical exam, a petechial rash is present all over his body. Suspecting meningitis, the physician orders a lumbar puncture, revealing gram-negative diplococci (*Neisseria meningitidis*) on Gram stain. The physician wishes to use a more sensitive test to confirm this as the causative agent. Which of the following tests combines features of gel diffusion and immunoelectrophoresis and is applicable only to negatively charged antigens?

a. Coagglutination (COA)
b. Counterimmunoelectrophoresis (CIE)
c. Enzyme-linked immunosorbent assay (ELISA)
d. Latex agglutination (LA)
e. Radioimmunoassay (RIA)

**487.** A 21-year old female presents to the emergency room with a high fever, hypotension, and a diffuse, macular, sunburn-like rash that is desquamating. She is also vomiting, has profuse diarrhea, leukocytosis, thrombocytopenia, and elevated BUN and creatinine levels. History from her room mate reveals that these symptoms started soon after the patient began packing her nose to stop chronic nose bleeds. Suspecting *Staphylococcus aureus,* a nasal swab specimen is obtained and sent to the lab. Which of the following rapid tests will be ordered and depends on the presence of protein A on certain strains of *S. aureus*?

a. Coagglutination (COA)
b. Counterimmunoelectrophoresis (CIE)
c. Enzyme-linked immunosorbent assay (ELISA)
d. Latex agglutination (LA)
e. Radioimmunoassay (RIA)

**488.** A 50-year-old building contractor arrives in your office complaining of abdominal pain that has increased in severity over the last 3 months. He has noticed melenic stool. Ordering a sigmoidoscopy, a 10-cm mass is visualized in the transverse colon. Surgery is immediately done and the tumor excised. As part of the patient's post surgical follow through of this resected carcinoma of the colon, blood is obtained and sent to the lab to monitor levels of the tumor marker known as Carcinoembryonic Antigen (CEA). Which of the following tests involves the measurement of very small quantities, of CEA, through competition of radiolabeled and unlabeled antigen for the same limited amount of antibody?

a. Coagglutination (COA)
b. Counterimmunoelectrophoresis (CIE)
c. Enzyme-linked immunosorbent assay (ELISA)
d. Latex agglutination (LA)
e. Radioimmunoassay (RIA)

**489.** A 13-year-old male arrives at his doctor's office with a severe sore throat and very high fever. On physical exam, the physician observes his pharynx to be inflamed with a significant exudate along with tender cervical lymph nodes. Labs reveal a leukocytosis. Suspecting Group A β-hemolytic *Streptococcus pyogenes* a throat swab and culture are obtained. Using a rapid diagnostic kit recently obtained, the physician decides to test the specimens himself. This test involves inert particles that are sensitized with either antigen or antibody. Which of the following tests is used extensively to detect microbial antigens rapidly (5 minutes or less)?

a. Coagglutination (COA)
b. Counterimmunoelectrophoresis (CIE)
c. Enzyme-linked immunosorbent assay (ELISA)
d. Latex agglutination (LA)
e. Radioimmunoassay (RIA)

**490.** A 7-month-old baby who is failing to thrive is brought into a neighborhood clinic. History reveals that the baby's mother died of AIDS 2 months ago. Blood is obtained and sent to the laboratory to check for HIV infection. The physician orders a test whose detection system is based on enzymatic activity. Which of the following tests is a heterogeneous immunoassay?

a. Coagglutination (COA)
b. Counterimmunoelectrophoresis (CIE)
c. Enzyme-linked immunosorbent assay (ELISA)
d. Latex agglutination (LA)
e. Radioimmunoassay (RIA)

### Item 491–495

A 29-year-old pregnant female gives birth to a stillborn child. History reveals that the woman continued to have close contact with her five cats, by emptying litter boxes and feeding them raw meat, during pregnancy, against her physician's advice. An autopsy is conducted, and multiple cysts are found in the fetal brain, lungs, liver, and eyes. As a confirmatory test, the pathologist orders an enzyme immunoassay to detect the presence of *Toxoplasma gondii*. The diagram below presents the various steps (labeled A–F) of the enzyme immunoassay.

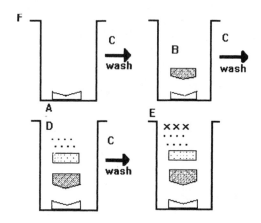

**491.** Failure of or improper methods for which step in the process is the primary cause of high background color?

a. A
b. B
c. C
d. D
e. E
f. F

**492.** Where is unlabeled antibody attached if this enzyme immunoassay is intended for detection of antigen?

a. A
b. B
c. C
d. D
e. E
f. F

**493.** What is the location of the "solid phase"?

a. A
b. B
c. C
d. D
e. E
f. F

**494.** Addition of reagent at which step will cause color in the positive control well and reactive patient specimens?

a. A
b. B
c. C
d. D
e. E
f. F

**495.** What is the location of the patient specimen in the diagram?

a.  A
b.  B
c.  C
d.  D
e.  E
f.  F

**496.** An 18-year-old male patient with acute lymphocytic leukemia fails all standard chemotherapies. Cells from an HLA-nonidentical donor are used to perform a bone marrow transplant. Prior to transplantation, the patient is given broad-spectrum antibiotics and an immunosuppressive regimen. Within 2–4 weeks, lymphocyte and granulocyte numbers begin to rise, confirming bone marrow cell engraftment. However, 1 month later, the patient develops diarrhea, jaundice, and a severe maculopapular rash. Physical exam reveals hepatomegaly and splenomegaly. Which of the following is most likely occurring?

a.  Acute rejection
b.  Chronic rejection
c.  Cyclosporine A toxicity
d.  Graft versus host disease (GVHD)
e.  Hyperacute rejection

**497.** A 27-year-old male patient (blood group O) arrives at the emergency room with a massive intestinal bleed (hematochezia). Within hours he has lost half of his blood volume, and you decide to transfuse. Due to human error, you transfuse blood, group AB, into him and within minutes, he develops a fever, chills, dyspnea, and a dramatic drop in blood pressure. This reaction is most likely due to which of the following?

a.  A cell-mediated response against AB antigens
b.  IgG production by the recipient in response to AB antigens
c.  Preformed anti-A and anti-B antibodies in the recipient
d.  Preformed anti-A and anti-B antibodies of the blood donor
e.  Preformed isohemagglutinins of the IgG isotype

**498.** During a clinic office visit, a 35-year-old male stockbroker shows signs of excessive nervousness and irritability and complains that the office is too hot. History and physical reveal the presence of a goiter and exophthalmia. Laboratory analysis of his blood reveals high antibody titers against the thyroid-stimulating hormone (TSH) receptor. Which of the following is the most likely diagnosis?

a.  Goodpasture's syndrome
b.  Graves' disease
c.  Hashimoto's disease
d.  Juvenile onset diabetes mellitus
e.  Myasthenia gravis
f.  Pernicious anemia
g.  Rheumatoid arthritis
h.  Systemic lupus erythematosus (SLE)

**499.** A 9-year-old female with a recent history of weight loss and vision problems arrives at the hospital. Soon after, it is determined that she has low blood glucose, and autoantibodies against β cells are detected in her serum. Which of the following is the most likely diagnosis?

a.  Goodpasture's syndrome
b.  Grave's disease
c.  Hashimoto's disease
d.  Juvenile onset diabetes mellitus
e.  Myasthenia gravis
f.  Pernicious anemia
g.  Rheumatoid arthritis
h.  Systemic lupus erythematosus (SLE)

**500.** A 35-year-old woman with fever, weight loss, fatigue, and painful joints and muscles presents to her physician's office. The physician notes that she has marked photosensitivity and a rash on the cheeks and over the bridge of her nose. Laboratory tests reveal anemic conditions and the presence of anti-DNA antibodies. Which of the following is the most likely diagnosis?

a.  Goodpasture's syndrome
b.  Graves' disease
c.  Hashimoto's disease
d.  Juvenile onset diabetes mellitus
e.  Myasthenia gravis
f.  Pernicious anemia
g.  Rheumatoid arthritis
h.  Systemic lupus erythematosus (SLE)

# Immunology

## Answers

**410–413. The answers are 410-a, 411-c, 412-c, 413-d.** *(Parslow, pp 197–202, 380, 386–388. Levinson, pp 445–452.)* Reactions to small amounts of drugs can occur, as illustrated in the skin test using penicilloyl-polylysine to reveal a penicillin allergy. The diagrams in 1, 2, 3, and 4 represent Type I, II, III, and IV hypersensitivity, respectively. The table below describes these reactions in detail.

| | **HYPERSENSITIVITY REACTIONS** | |
| **Mediator** | **Type** | **Reaction** |
| --- | --- | --- |
| Antibody (IgE) | I (immediate, anaphylactic) | IgE antibody is induced by allergen and binds to mast cells and basophils. When exposed to the allergen again, the allergen cross-links the bound IgE, which induces degranulation and release of mediators, e.g., histamine. |
| Antibody (IgG) | II (cytotoxic) | Antigens on a cell surface combine with antibody; this leads to complement-mediated lysis, e.g., transfusion or Rh reactions, or autoimmune hemolytic anemia. |
| Antibody (IgG) | III (immune complex) | Antigen-antibody immune complexes are deposited in tissues, complement is activated, and polymorphonuclear cells are attracted to the site. They release lysosomal enzymes, causing tissue damage. |
| Cell | IV (delayed) | Helper T lymphocytes sensitized by an antigen release lymphokines upon second contact with the same antigen. The lymphokines induce inflammation and activate macrophages, which, in turn, release various mediators. |

*Reprinted, with permission, from Levinson W, Jawetz E. Medical Microbiology, 7e. New York: McGraw-Hill, 2002:415.*

**414–415. The answers are 414-b, 415-a.** *(Parslow, pp 117, 302–305. Levinson, pp 431, 432, 463–465.)* Bruton's agammaglobulinemia is a congenital defect that becomes apparent at approximately 6 months of age, when maternal IgG is diminished. It occurs in males and is characterized by a defective *btk* gene, very small tonsils, low levels of all five classes of immunoglobulins, and no mature B cells. Thus, the child is unable to produce immunoglobulins and develops a series of bacterial infections characterized by recurrences and progression to more serious infections such as septicemia. The most common organisms responsible for infection are *H. influenzae* and *S. pneumoniae*. Cell-mediated immunity is not affected, and the child is able to respond normally to diseases that require this immune response for resolution. Treatment consists of pooled IgG.

*Note:* Immunodeficiency is characterized by unusual and recurrent infections:

- B cell (antibody) deficiency—bacterial infections
- T cell deficiency—viral, fungal, and protozoal infections
- Phagocytic cell deficiency—pyogenic infections (bacterial), skin infections, systemic bacterial opportunistic infections
- Complement deficiencies—pyogenic infections (bacterial)

**416–417. The answers are 416-e, 417-a.** *(Levinson, pp 393–401.)* Cells can be differentiated based on unique cell surface markers (antigens). In this case, a CD4:CD8 ratio of less than 1 indicates a significant reduction in the Helper T lymphocyte population. The surface proteins that best represent this pool are MHC I, TCR, CD3, and CD28. CD4 is also associated with Helper T lymphocytes. B lymphocytes have MHC I, IgM, B7 CD19, and CD20. Cytotoxic T lymphocytes have MHC I, TCR, CD3, and CD8, while macrophages have MHC I, MHC II, abd CD14. An important fact to remember is that all healthy cells other than mature red cells have class I MHC. The B7 surface protein on the antigen presenting cell (B cell) is the costimulatory molecule and must interact with the CD28 on the helper T cell for full activation to occur. (See the figures.)

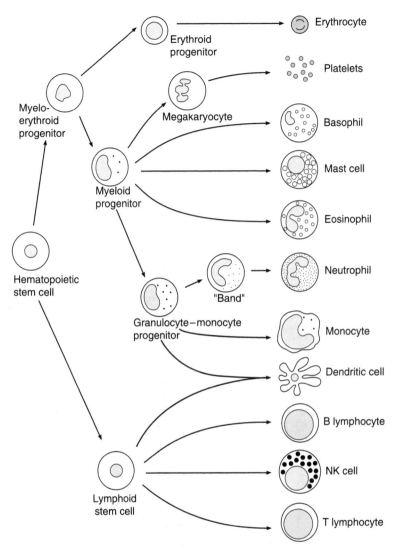

Schematic overview of hematopoiesis, emphasizing the erythroid, myeloid, and lymphoid pathways. This highly simplified depiction omits many recognized intermediate cell types in each pathway. All of the cells shown here develop to maturity in the bone marrow, except T lymphocytes, which develop from marrow-derived progenitors that migrate to the thymus. A common lymphoid stem cell serves as the progenitor of T and B lymphocytes and of natural killer (NK) cells. Dendritic cells arise from both the myeloid and lymphoid lineages. (*Reproduced, with permission, from Parslow TG et al. Medical Immunology, 10e. New York: McGraw-Hill, 2001: 3.*)

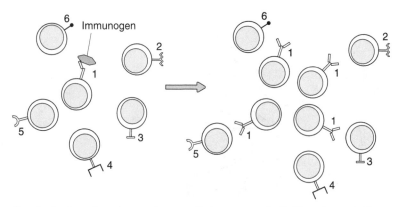

Clonal selection of lymphocytes by a specific immunogen. **Left:** The unimmunized lymphocyte population is composed of cells from many different clones, each with its own antigen specificity, indicated here by the distinctive shapes of the surface antigen receptors. **Right:** Contact with an immunogen leads to selective proliferation (positive selection) of any clone or clones that can recognize that specific immunogen. *(Reproduced, with permission, from Parslow TG et al. Medical Immunology, 10e. New York: McGraw-Hill, 2001:62.)*

**418. The answer is a.** *(Parslow, pp 79–80, 700–703. Levinson, pp 92, 160.)* Recurrent severe infection is an indication for clinical evaluation of immune status. Live vaccines, including BCG attenuated from *M. tuberculosis*, should not be used in the evaluation of a patient's immune competence because patients with severe immunodeficiencies may develop an overwhelming infection (disseminated disease) from the vaccine. For the same reason, oral (Sabin) polio vaccine is not advisable for use in such persons.

**419. The answer is e.** *(Parslow, p 625. Levinson, p 309.)* Measles-like virus has been isolated from the brain cells of patients with SSPE. The role of the host immune response in the causation of SSPE has been supported by several findings including the following: (1) progression of disease despite high levels of humoral antibody; (2) presence of a factor that blocks lymphocyte-mediated immunity to SSPE-measles virus in SSPE-cerebrospinal fluid (CSF); (3) lysis of brain cells from SSPE patients by SSPE serum or CSF in the presence of complement (a similar mechanism could cause in vivo tissue injury). SSPE is particularly common in those who acquired measles before 2 years of age and is very rare after measles vaccination.

Higher-than-normal levels of serum antibodies (Ab) to measles virus and local synthesis of measles Ab in CSF, as evidenced by the oligoclonal IgG, imply a connection between the virus and multiple sclerosis (MS). However, the other studies have implicated the other viruses. Several studies of cell-mediated hypersensitivity to measles and other viruses in MS have been done, but the results have been conflicting. Definite conclusions regarding defects in cellular immunity in this disease cannot be reached until further research is completed.

**420. The answer is c.** (*Parslow, pp 84–85, 275. Levinson, p 428.*) Transplantation terminology is being tested in this question. An autograft is a transfer of an individual's own tissue to another site in the body. An isograft (syngeneic graft) is the transfer of tissue between genetically identical individuals. An allograft is the transfer of tissue between genetically different members of the same species. While a xenograft is the transfer of tissue between different species. In this case, one unit is the patient's own blood (an autologous donation) while the second unit is his brother's blood (most like an allograft donation). If his brother had been a twin then (e) would be the correct answer.

**421. The answer is e.** (*Parslow, pp 251–252. Levinson, p 56, 422–423.*) The graph presented in the question exhibits hemagglutinating antibody responses to primary and secondary immunization with any standard antigen. Curve B represents the early response to primary immunization, which is chiefly an IgM response. Rechallenge elicits an accelerated response that mainly involves IgG and occurs 2–5 days after reimmunization. IgM has a molecular weight of 900,000 and is a pentamer that the fetus can produce quite early in gestation. IgM (and IgG) have the ability to activate complement, appear along with sIgD as the B cell receptor on B lymphocytes, and like IgA require J chains to join the Fc chains of each monomer together.

**422. The answer is b.** (*Parslow, pp 215–217. Levinson, pp 451, 455, 458–459.*) This clinical case represents a patient suffering with Systemic Lupus Erythematosus (SLE). The diagnosis of SLE is best supported by detecting the presence of anti-dsDNA and anti-Smith (anti-Sm) antibodies. The presence of anti-dsDNA antibodies are very specific for SLE and represent a poor prognosis for disease. Antinuclear antibodies (ANA) can also be detected using fluorescent antibody tests.

**423. The answer is a.** (*Parslow, pp 221–223. Levinson, pp 65, 117–118, 227, 437–438, 439.*) ELISA (enzyme-linked immunosorbent assay) methods can be used to detect either antigens or antibodies. If antigen is to be detected, then specific antibody is initially bound to the plate (see A in the diagram presented with the question). If antibody is to be detected, then antigen is bound to the solid phase. The bound antigen and antibody then "captures" the analyte to be detected. One of the major causes for high background in ELISA tests is the failure to wash off unbound antigen or antibody (see B in the diagram presented with the question). ELISA is routinely used to screen patient sera for different antibodies (including anti–HIV-1 antibodies). In this case, the well is initially coated with HIV-1 antigen, and the patient sera is tested for anti–HIV-1 antibodies.

**424. The answer is a.** (*Parslow, pp 216, 218. Levinson, pp 436–438.*) In the Ouchterlony agar-gel diffusion test, an antigen and a series of antibodies (or an antibody and a series of antigens) are allowed to diffuse toward each other. At the zone of optimal proportions of the reactants, a precipitin line occurs. Cross-reactions between antigens or antibodies tested can be detected by (1) a shortening of the major precipitin band contiguous to the cross-reacting substance, or (2) the identity of precipitin reaction between the two cross-dressing substances. The figures presented in the question illustrate both types of cross-reaction. In the first bleed pattern shown in the question, cross-reaction between antigen X and antigen A is recognizable only by a shortening of the precipitin band between the center well and X on the A well side (relative to the band going directly into the normal saline well). In the second bleed pattern, full cross-reaction of X and A is apparent. No other cross-reactions are seen.

**425. The answer is a.** (*Parslow, p 334. Levinson, pp 55, 57, 463–467.*) The patient in this case has chronic granulomatous disease (CGD), an X-linked (65%) or autosomal recessive (35%) inherited disease. Patients with CGD are not able to generate a respiratory burst after granulocyte and monocyte stimulation. Thus, they are unable to kill microorganisms. Answers a, b, and c are all involved in the respiratory burst; however, the central enzyme is the NADPH oxidase (answer a). Without this enzyme, hydrogen peroxide (answer b), superoxide (answer c), and other microbial reactive oxygen species would not be generated.

**426. The answer is b.** *(Parslow, pp 113–114. Levinson, pp 418–421, 463–468.)* Immunoglobulin gene rearrangement errors can contribute to the development of many types of leukemia and lymphoma. Some genetic alterations are characteristic of particular histologic entities: t(8;14) in Burkitt's lymphoma, t(14;18) in follicular lymphoma, t(11;14) in mantle cell lymphoma, and t(2;5) in anaplastic large cell lymphoma.

**427. The answer is c.** *(Parslow, pp 82–83. Levinson, p 395–400.)* The figure shown in the question is a schematic representation of the MHC Class I molecule, which has a CD8 binding site ($\alpha$3) and a peptide-binding site ($\alpha$1 and $\alpha$2). MHC Class I is active on all nucleated cells.

**428. The answer is a.** *(Parslow, pp 101–102. Levinson, pp 413–417.)* The initial response to a new infection is with an IgM class antibody. IgM develops quickly and usually disappears within a few months. The secondary response is IgG and reflects the patient's immune status or, in the case of chickenpox, a vaccination given.

**429–431. The answers are 429-e, 430-a, 431-a.** *(Levinson, pp 313–321, 437–441.)* A male patient with the presentation as outlined in question 429 (fatigue, weight loss, and lymphadenopathy) must be tested for antibodies to HIV. While other antibody tests may be relevant after the primary diagnosis, they must be considered after HIV is ruled out. Certainly, infectious mononucleosis is a possibility, but its occurrence in this age group is not as frequent as HIV. Patients are tested first by an ELISA screening test. If this test is positive (X2), then a confirmatory Western blot is performed. A Western blot separates the immune response into antibody production for specific components of the virus, that is, envelope, gag, and so forth. The following table shows the various bands that could be seen on a widely used Western blot and their identification by specific antigen source. There are at least three schemes for interpreting Western blots. Assuming technical competence in the laboratory, one of the more common reasons for falsely positive ELISAs and Western blots is an influenza vaccination within the past few months. A rare patient may have antibody to the cell line used to grow virus. Unlike Lyme disease, there is no reported cross-reactivity with Epstein-Barr virus (EBV) or HTLV. There appears to be no naturally occurring antibody to retroviruses.

| Antigen | Source |
|---|---|
| gp 160 | Env gene product |
| gp 120 | Env fragment |
| gp 41 | Transmembrane fragment |
| gp 31 | |
| gp 51 | Pol gene product |
| p 66 | |
| p 24 | Core protein (gag) |

*Abbreviations:* gp, glycoprotein; p, protein; env, envelope; pol, polymerase.

**432. The answer is d.** (*Parslow, p 344. Levinson, p 433.*) Patients with complement deficiencies such as C5 through C9, which form the membrane attack complex (MAC), are predisposed to disseminated meningococcal (neisserial) disease. These patients may also be susceptible to gonococcal (neisserial) infection. There appears to be no disposition to AIDS or to fungal, parasitic, or pneumococcal infections.

**433. The answer is d.** (*Parslow, pp 23–24. Levinson, pp 430, 455–460.*) The acute-phase response is a primitive, nonspecific defense reaction, mediated by the liver, that increases innate immunity and other protective functions in stressful times. It can be triggered by chronic autoimmune disorders such as rheumatoid arthritis and Crohn's disease. This response occurs when hepatocytes are exposed to IL-6 and IL-1 of TNF-α. LPS is a potent inducer of these cytokines. They are responsible for fever, somnolence, loss of appetite, and, if the response is prolonged, anemia and cachexia (wasting). A traditional assay known as the *erythrocyte sedimentation rate* (ESR) may be used as an indicator of an acute-phase response. The ESR involves measuring the rate at which the red blood cells fall through plasma, which increases as fibrinogen concentration rises. Currently, Crohn's disease may be treated with infusions of a drug known as infliximab which is a mouse-human chimeric antibody against human TNF-α.

**434. The answer is d.** (*Parslow, p 703. Levinson, pp 390, 413–418.*) Maternal transfer of antibody (secretory IgA in the colostrum of breast milk), however, is passive but still confers specific immunity. It is termed *passive acquired* immunity. Natural immunity is nonspecific. The natural immune functions described are not specific for a certain antigen. For example, certain proteins such as C-reactive protein (CRP) are acute-phase reactants. While elevated CRP is seen in infection, it is not disease-specific.

**435. The answer is b.** (*Parslow, pp 76–77. Levinson, pp 390–391.*) Haptens (incomplete antigens) are not themselves antigenic, but when coupled to a cell or carrier protein become antigenic and induce antibodies that can bind the hapten alone (in the absence of the carrier protein). They are small molecules that are generally less than 1000 Da. While haptens react with antibodies, they are not immunogenic because they do not activate T cells and cannot bind the MHC. Haptens are significant in disease; penicillin is a hapten and can cause severe life-threatening allergic reaction by destruction of erythrocytes. Catechols in the oils of poison ivy plants are haptens and cause a significant skin inflammatory response. Chloramphenicol is a hapten that can lead to the destruction of leukocytes and cause agranulocytosis. Sedormid is a hapten that can cause thrombocytopenia and purpura (bleeding) through the destruction of platelets.

**436. The answer is e.** (*Levinson, pp 65, 435–441.*) The radial immunodiffusion and immunoelectrophoresis are two tests used to evaluate humoral immunity. Evaluating humoral immunity consists of measuring the levels of IgM, IgG, and IgA in the patient's serum. Whereas total IgG is greater than total IgM in the fetus due to the maternal transfer of IgG and not IgM across the placenta, it is important to remember that IgM is the antibody produced in the greatest amounts by the fetus. The fetus also produces IgG and IgA, but the fetus produces greater amounts of IgM than these other two important antibodies.

**437. The answer is b.** (*Parslow, pp 95–97, 101. Ryan, pp 124–127. Levinson, pp 413–421.*) The hinge region consists mostly of cysteine and proline residues, allowing for the formation of interchain disulphide bonds and flexibility, respectively. There appears to be considerable flexibility in the hinge region between the Fc and the two F(ab) portions of the molecule. This allows the molecule to assume either a T shape or a Y shape. The two arms of the antibody are identical and possess the same paratopes; hence, they will recognize identical epitopes. Each variable and constant heavy and light chains consist of the same amino acid sequences. IgG is the most abundant antibody in the serum. It migrates in the gamma-globulin fraction during serum protein separation and composes 80% of the antibody concentration in the serum. Two enzymes, papain and pepsin, can digest an IgG antibody molecule by cleaving (hydrolysis) the antibody molecule on the N and C terminus sides, respectively, of the sulfhydryl bridge binding the heavy chains. Finally, antibodies protect the host by neutralization (preventing adherence), opsonizing (promoting phagocytosis), and activating complement (lysis). (See the figure.)

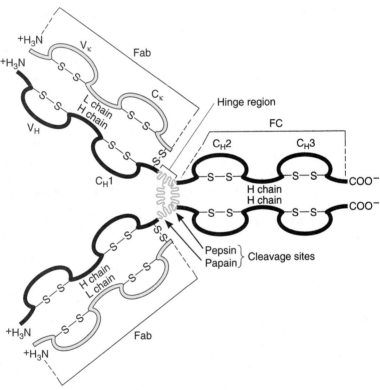

Schematic model of an IgG1 (κ) human antibody molecule showing the basic four-chain structure and domains ($V_H$, $C_H1$, etc.). Sites of enzymatic cleavage by pepsin and papain are shown. (*Reproduced, with permission, from Parslow TG et al.* Medical Immunology, *10e. New York: McGraw-Hill, 2001: 96.*)

**438. The answer is d.** (*Parslow, p 637. Levinson, pp 313–321.*) HIV-2 disease is very rare in the United States. However, HIV-2 is present in Africa, the Far East, and some parts of the Caribbean. Many of the screening tests for HIV-1 will not detect antibodies to HIV-2. Either a separate HIV-2 antibody test or a combination HIV-1/2 is necessary. While HTLV disease is also seen in the same geographic areas, the symptoms displayed by this patient are more akin to HIV disease. While an HIV-1 RNA PCR is a useful test for monitoring the results of HIV therapy, it is not approved for diagnosis, nor will it detect HIV-2 nucleic acid.

**439. The answer is c.** (*Parslow, pp 143–144, 146. Levinson, pp 407–408.*) NK cells do not express a cell surface TCR/CD3 complex and are CD4−. About half of human NK cells are CD8+. Also, most NK cells express an Fc IgG receptor, known as CD16, and CD56, a neural cell adhesion molecule variant. NK cells are generally CD16+, CD56+, and CD3−, which contrasts them with T cells which are CD3+, CD16−, and CD56−.

**440. The answer is e.** (*Parslow, pp 175, 183–184. Levinson, pp 53–56, 431. Ryan, p 49.*) C3a and C5a are potent mediators of inflammation; that is, they have anaphylatoxic activity. This activity is characterized by smooth-muscle contraction and the degranulation of mast cells and basophils leading to the release of histamine and other vasoactive substances, causing increased vascular (capillary) permeability. C5a is the most potent of these anaphylatoxins; however, it also serves another role as a potent chemotactic agent, attracting polymorphonucleated neutrophils and macrophages to the site of inflammation.

**441. The answer is d.** (*Jawetz, pp 350–351. Levinson, pp 221–223. Parslow, pp 160–161.*) Alpha and beta interferons are proteins that can induce an antiviral state in uninfected cells via the production of secondary protein factors that inhibit viral protein synthesis by degrading only viral mRNA (not host mRNA). Also, they can increase the expression of MHC Class I proteins, which enable an infected cell to present viral antigens and facilitate killing by CTLs, and they can stimulate the production of gamma interferon. In addition, gamma interferon increases MHC Class II expression and antigen presentation in all cells and activates NK cells to kill virus-infected cells. Interferons have no direct effect on extracellular virus particles.

**442. The answer is a.** (*Parslow, p 721. Levinson, pp 426–430.*) Allograft rejection is primarily a T cell response to foreign tissue. Many immunosuppressive measures exist, including cyclosporine, tacrolimus, sirolimus, azathioprine, monoclonal antibodies, radiation, and corticosteroids. Commonly used, the corticosteroids reduce inflammatory response and are generally administered by cytotoxic drugs, such as cyclosporine. Corticosteroids function as immunosuppressive agents by inhibiting cytokine production, such as IL-1 and TNF, and also by lysing certain T cell types. Lymphoid irradiation is usually done so that the bone marrow is shielded. This removes lymphocytes from lymph nodes and spleen while allowing the patient to have the capacity to regenerate new T and B cells. Likewise, antilymphocyte globulin will destroy the recipient's lymphocytes, especially T cells. Destruction of donor B cells and T cells would not play a role in the immunosuppression of the graft recipient. In graft crises, monoclonal antibody to CD3 is sometimes given. This targets mature T lymphocytes for destruction.

**443. The answer is c.** (*Levinson, pp 91–94, 422–423.*) With repeated immunization, higher titers of all antibodies are observed, and, as priming is repeated, the immune response recruits B cells of progressively greater affinity. The affinity of antibody for a hapten-protein complex rises, cross-reactivity also rises, and the response becomes wider in specificity. As the number of antigenic sites detected per reacting particle increases, the avidity increases. In addition to shifts in the class of immunoglobulin synthesized in response to an antigen (IgM to IgG), shifts also may occur in the idiotype of antibody.

**444. The answer is c.** (*Levinson, pp 435–438.*) In precipitation reactions, both the antigen and the antibody are soluble. The antibody cross-links antigen molecules, creating an increasing lattice that eventually forms an insoluble precipitate. The antigen must be divalent, and the antigen/antibody proportion is critical in order for detectable precipitate to form. The prozone is the zone of antibody excess. The postzone is the zone of antigen excess. The zone of equivalence is the zone where the proportion of antibody and antigen is optimal for precipitate formation. Titer is the reciprocal of the highest dilution (ratio) of antibody (or antigen) at which there is still a detectable reaction. (See figure below.)

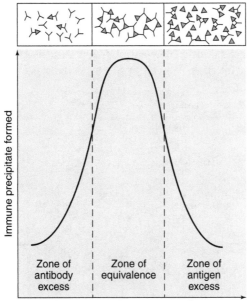

Zone of antibody excess | Zone of equivalence | Zone of antigen excess

Increasing antigen concentration

Immune precipitate formed

*Modified and reproduced, with permission, from Stites D, Terr A, Parslow T (eds.) Basic and Clinical Immunology, 9e. Originally published by Appleton & Lange. Copyright © 1997 by The McGraw-Hill Companies.)*

**445. The answer is b.** *(Parslow, pp 207–209. Levinson, pp 414–419.)* Each secretory IgA molecule has a molecular weight of 400,000 and consists of two H2L2 units and one molecule each of J chain and secretory component. Some IgA exists in serum as a monomer H2L2 with a molecular weight of 160,000. Some bacteria, such as *Neisseria,* can destroy IgA-1 by producing protease. It is the major immunoglobulin in milk, saliva, tears, mucus, sweat, gastric fluid, and colostrum. IgA does not fix complement, so one would anticipate that a complement fixation test would not be useful for IgA antibody.

**446. The answer is d.** *(Parslow, pp 380–383. Levinson, pp 431–434.)* Both IgG and IgM activate complement by the classic pathway, while IgA activates it by the alternative pathway. IgA, IgD, and IgE cannot activate complement. Complement is a system of several proteins that is activated by either an immune or a nonimmune pathway. Both of these pathways result in the production of many biologically active components that cause cell lysis and death. In this clinical case, the patient is suffering from severe liver failure. This significant reduction in liver function has led to a reduced ability by the patient to produce sufficient complement proteins, and as a result the patient is predisposed to infections caused by pyogenic bacteria. See the figure below.

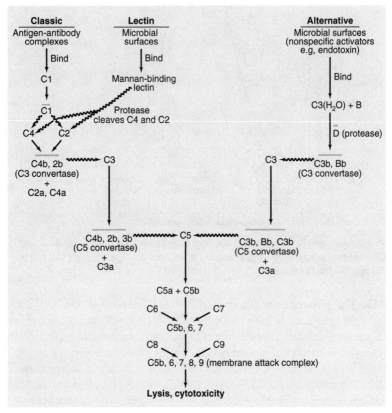

The classic and alternative pathways of the complement system. ⟿ indicates that proteolytic cleavage of the molecule at the tip of the arrow has occurred; a line over a complex indicates that it is enzymatically active. Note that the nomenclature of the cleavage products of C2 is undecided. Some call the large fragment C2a and others call it C2b. The C3 convertase is depicted here as C4b,2b. Note that proteases associated with the mannose-binding lectin cleave C4 as well as C2. (*Reprinted, with permission, from Levinson W, Jawetz E. Medical Microbiology and Immunology, 7e. New York: McGraw-Hill, 2002:401.*)

**447–451. The answers are 447-d, 448-c, 449-e, 450-b, 451-a.**
*(Parslow, pp 95–114. Levinson, pp 413–424, 423, 463–468.)* IgG antibody provides an "immune history." That is, IgG antibody persists in most people and indicates the antigens to which they have been exposed. IgG is not formed early in infection but is a secondary response arising weeks to months after antigenic challenge. IgG also has a built-in memory. Even people with very low levels of specific IgG will respond to an antigen challenge with an IgG response.

IgM antibody, in contrast, arises early in infection and then disappears within a couple of months. IgM is intravascular and does not cross the placental barrier. For this reason, infants with specific IgG responses to disease must be tested for IgM to determine whether their immune systems have produced antibody or whether the test was positive because of passively transferred IgG. The clinical case described in question 448 is of a young patient with Hyper-IgM syndrome. This immune deficiency presents early in life with severe pyogenic infections, resembling those seen in X-linked hypogammaglobulinemia; however, unlike X-linked hypogammaglobulinemia (very low levels of all immunoglobulins, virtual absence of B cells, found in young boys with female carriers being immunolgically normal), Hyper-IgM syndrome patients have a high IgM concentration, low IgG, IgA, and IgE concentration, and normal T and B cell numbers. The problem exists in a mutational defect in the CD40 ligand in CD4-positive helper T cells leading to failure of normal interaction between this ligand on T cells and CD40 on B cell surfaces. This failure leads to an inability of the B cells to class switch from IgM production to other antibodies. Treatment includes pooled gamma-globulin.

IgA antibody is involved in local immunity at the level of the mucous membrane. IgA antibody also arises early in disease. IgA antibody is short-lived and will disappear similarly to IgM.

IgE antibody is characteristically seen in parasitic infections, particularly worm (helminth) infections because of the attraction of eosinophils to the site of the infestation. Certain allergies are due to excessive production of IgE. The patient in this case has Trichinosis as a result of consuming undercooked pork and ingesting *Trichinella spiralis*. IgE specific for worm proteins binds to receptors on eosinophils promoting the release of worm destroying enzymes involved in the antibody-dependent cellular cytotoxicity (ADCC) response.

IgD antibody consists of two light chains and two heavy chains. Its role is not known, but it can be found on the surface of lymphocytes, where it may act as a surface receptor.

IgG is susceptible to proteolytic enzymes, which may explain why it is present in such low levels in serum. In addition, the fetus has more total IgG, than IgM, as a result of maternal placental IgG transfer, even though IgM is produced in greater amounts by the fetus.

**452–456. The answers are 452-a, 453-b, 454-e, 455-c, 456-d.**
*(Parslow, p 692. Levinson pp 245–249, 257–258, 291–292, 309.)* B. burgdorferi, the causative agent of Lyme disease, elicits an acute antibody response. IgM appears within days to a few weeks following tick bite, and IgG appears a few weeks later. IgG persists; IgM does not. Cross-reactions occur with other treponemes.

Fifth disease is a viral exanthem commonly seen in children 8–12-years-old. Children are ill for a few days but recover without incident, usually within about 1 week. Unfortunately, if a pregnant female acquires the disease in the first trimester of pregnancy, the fetus is at risk. The causative agent is thought to be a Parvovirus (Parvovirus B19). Fifth disease is also known as erythema infectiosum or Slapped Cheek syndrome. The four other maculopapular or macular rash diseases of childhood are measles, roseola, rubella, and scarlet fever.

Adults with no titer to varicella (VZV) are at risk for acquisition of chickenpox. If they are health care workers, there is additional risk in transmitting VZV to immunodeficient children. Antibodies to VZV are readily detected by both enzyme immunoassay (EIA) and fluorescent antibody (FA) techniques.

Delta agent is a recently discovered antigen associated with HBsAg. Its presence usually correlates with HBsAg chronic carriers who have chronic active hepatitis. EIA and radioimmunoassay (RIA) tests are available to detect antibodies to delta agent.

SSPE is thought to be caused by a measles-related virus present in the central nervous system. Most SSPE patients show elevated measles virus antibodies in serum and CSF. In patients with multiple sclerosis (MS), lower CSF antibody titers have been observed, suggesting a possible etiologic role for measles virus in MS.

**457–461. The answers are 457-d, 458-c, 459-d, 460-b, 461-d.**
*(Levinson, pp 122, 463–468.)* Immunodeficiency disorders can be categorized according to whether the defect primarily involves humoral immunity (bone marrow-derived, or B lymphocytes) or cellular immunity

(thymus-derived, or T lymphocytes) or both. Swiss-type hypogammaglobulinemia, ataxia-telangiectasia, the Wiskott-Aldrich syndrome, and severe combined immunodeficiency disorders all involve defective B cell and T cell function. Infantile X-linked agammaglobulinemia is caused chiefly by deficient B cell activity, whereas thymic hypoplasia is mainly a T cell immunodeficiency disorder.

In Question 457, this 2-year-old patient has ataxia (staggering)-telangiectasia, (spider angiomas), an autosomal recessive immune disorder associated with both a lymphopenia (cellular) and IgA deficiency (humoral). Question 458 describes a patient with X-linked hypogammaglobulinemia or Bruton's agammaglobulinemia which only occurs in boys and is characterized by low levels of all immunoglobulin classes and the absence of almost all B cells. Pre-B cells are present; however, they fail to differentiate into B cells. Cell-mediated immunity is relatively normal. Recurrent bacterial infections occur after about 6 months of age when protective maternal IgG antibody declines. The fetus represented in Question 459 has severe combined immunodeficiency disease (SCID) characterized by defects in early stem-cell differentiation. As a result B cells and T cells are both defective, immunoglobulins are very low, and tonsils and lymph nodes are absent. Thymic Aplasia or DiGeorge syndrome marks the young child in Question 460. Failed development of the thymus and the parathyroids lead to hypoparathyroidism, hypocalcemia and ultimately a spastic paralysis (strong muscle contractions or tetany). Finally, Wiskott-Aldrich syndrome (Question 461), an X-linked defect, is associated with reduced IgM levels and variable cellular-mediated immunity.

**462–465. The answers are 462-a, 463-b, 464-c, 465-d.** *(Levinson, pp 426–430.)* Transplantation from one region of a person to another region of that same person is an *autograft* and has the best chance of succeeding. When a transplant is done between monozygotic twins, it is an *isograft* and has a complete MHC compatibility and a good chance of success. *Allografts* are between members of the same species, and *xenografts* are between members of different species. Both of these transplants have a high rate of rejection unless immunosuppression accompanies the transplant.

**466–468. The answers are 466-d, 467-c, 468-b.** *(Levinson, pp 415, 417–418, 423.)* Isotypes are determined by antigens of the immunoglobulin classes found in all individuals of one species. In addition to heavy-chain isotypes of IgA, IgD, IgE, IgG, and IgM, two light-chain isotypes exist for κ and λ chains.

Allotypes are differentiated by antigenic determinants that vary among individuals within a species and are recognized by cross-immunization of individuals in a species. Allotypes include the Gm marker of IgG and the Inv marker of light chains.

Idiotypes are antigenic determinants that appear only on the F(ab) fragments of antibodies and appear to be localized at the ligand-binding site; thus, anti-idiotype antisera may block reactions with the appropriate hapten. The carbohydrate side chains of immunoglobulins are relatively nonimmunogenic. New determinants may be exposed after papain cleavage of immunoglobulins, but these determinants are not included in the classification of the native molecule.

**469. The answer is f.** (*Parslow, pp 376–379. Levinson, pp 464–465.*) This patient has a classic case of hereditary angioedema. This disease is characterized by a deficiency of complement control proteins such as C1 esterase inhibitor, leading to overactive complement (reduced C4 levels). Uncontrolled generation of vasoactive peptides (C3a and C5a) causes increased blood vessel permeability, causing hereditary angioedema. Edema, especially of the larynx, obstructs the airways. Abdominal pain may indicate that the patient has angioedema of the gut.

**470. The answer is d.** (*Parslow, pp 569–571. Harrison's, pp 439, 530–531. Levinson, pp 461–462.*) The best-characterized human tumor-associated antigens are the oncofetal antigens. Carcinoembryonic antigen (CEA) is a glycoprotein and member of the immunoglobulin gene superfamily and is elevated in colorectal cancer. α-Fetoprotein (AFP) is analogous to albumin and elevated in hepatocellular carcinoma. Prostate-specific antigen (PSA) is elevated in prostatic cancer. CEA, AFP, and PSA are all glycoproteins. Melena refers to altered (black) blood per rectum, indicative of an upper gastrointestinal bleed.

**471–472. The answers are 471-b, 472-e.** (*Parslow, pp 636, 638–642.*) HIV infection affects mainly the immune system and the brain. The main immunologic feature of HIV infection is progressive depletion of the CD4 subset of T lymphocytes (T helper cells), causing a reversal in the normal CD4:CD8 ratio, leading to immunodeficiency. Currently, ELISA is the basic screening test to detect anti-HIV antibodies. Repeated reactive ELISA tests should be confirmed using either Western blot or immunofluorescence. The Western blot detects specific antibodies against the various HIV proteins (antigens).

**473. The answer is b.** (*Levinson, pp 410–413. Parslow, pp 251, 252, 257.*) Anti-Rh antibodies (IgG are reactive at 37°C) are the leading cause of hemolytic disease of the newborn (HDN). Currently, Rh immunization can be suppressed in antepartum or postpartem Rh− women if high-titer anti-Rh immunoglobulin (RhIg) is administered within 72 hours after the potentially sensitizing dose of Rh+ cells (i.e., the birth of the child).

**474–475. The answers are 474-g, 475-c.** (*Parslow, pp 320–321.*) Immune deficiency disorders occur as a result of impaired function in one or more of the major immune system components such as B lymphocytes, T lymphocytes, B and T lymphocytes, phagocytic cells, and complement. Unusual and recurrent infections are the hallmark of immunodeficiency. SCID occurs as a result of an early defect in stem cell differentiation and may be caused as a result of defective IL-2 receptors, adenosine deaminase deficiency, or failure to make MHC Class II antigens. This condition is characterized by B and T cell deficiency and presents with recurrent infections. The other disorders listed do not have both B and T cell deficiency with an absence of a thymus gland. Definitive treatment of SCID consists of stem cell transplantation, with the ideal donor being a sibling with identical human leukocyte antigens (HLA).

**476. The answer is b.** (*Parslow, pp 575–576, 699–700, 703–706.*) There are three forms of immunity: active, passive, and adoptive. Active immunity involves an individual making his or her own antibodies either naturally, by infection, or artificially, by immunizations. Passive immunity refers to the transfer of preformed antibodies from one individual to another either naturally (transplacental or enteromammary antibodies from mother to fetus) or artificially through gamma-globulin injections such as antitoxins, anti-Rh, and antivenoms (black widow spider bites and the like). Finally, adoptive immunity refers to the transfer of lymphoid cells from an actively immunized donor and does not involve antibody transfer.

**477. The answer is e.** (*Harrison's, pp 1918–1920, 1942–1943.*) Patients with T-cell defects are generally susceptible to viral, fungal, and protozoan

infections. This can be especially visible in patients with primary immunodeficiency diseases such as SCID. For further explanation of immunodeficiencies, please refer to the answer explanations for questions 414–415,
457–461, 474–475.

**478–479. The answers are 478-c, 479-b.** *(Parslow, p 217. Levinson,
pp 166–167, 438–440. Ryan, p 245.)* The complement fixation (CF) test is a
two-stage test. The first stage involves the union of antigen with its specific
antibody, followed by the fixation of complement to the antigen-antibody
structure. In order to determine whether complement has been "fixed," an
indicator system must be employed to determine the presence of free complement. Free complement binds to the complexes formed when red blood
cells (RBCs) are mixed with anti-RBC antibody; this binding causes lysis of
the cells. Complement that has been fixed before addition of RBCs and
anti-RBC antibody cannot cause lysis.

**480. The answer is b.** *(Parslow, pp 201–202, 370–372. Levinson, pp 445–448.)*
This is an example of a type I hypersensitivity reaction. Type I hypersensitivity is also referred to as anaphylaxis or immediate-type hypersensitivity. Major
components include IgE, mast cells/basophils, and pharmacologically active
mediators. Exposure to antigen causes IgE production, followed by sensitization of mast cells and basophils. Subsequent encounter with the same allergen
(antigen) leads to chemical mediator release (histamine and the like) and also
leads to clinical symptoms associated with asthma, allergic rhinitis, and so on.
This reaction can occur within minutes and can be extremely severe and life-
threatening.

**481–485. The answers are 481-c, 482-a, 483-b, 484-e, 485-d.**
*(Parslow, pp 628–630. Levinson, pp 283–292. Ryan, pp 541–553.)* The following
table presents the patterns of hepatitis B virus serologic markers observed
in various stages of infection with HBV. The diagnosis of HBV infection is
usually based on three tests: hepatitis B surface antigen, antibodies to surface antigen, and antibodies to core antigen. Tests are available, however, for
e antigen and antibodies to e antigen. A variety of testing methods are available and include enzyme immunoassay, radioimmunoassay, hemagglutination, latex agglutination, and immune adherence. The delta agent has
recently been described. The delta agent exacerbates infection with HBV,
apparently in a synergistic manner. Commercial tests are now available for
the delta agent.

| Interpretation | Serologic Markers | | | | | |
|---|---|---|---|---|---|---|
| | HBsAg | Anti-HBeAg | IgM Anti-HBc | Total Anti-HBc | Anti-HBe | HBs |
| Acute infection | | | | | | |
|   Incubation period | +* | +* | − | − | − | − |
|   Acute phase | + | + | + | + | − | − |
|   Early convalescent phase | + | − | + | + | + | − |
|   Convalescent phase | − | − | + | + | + | − |
|   Late convalescent phase | − | − | −† | + | + | + |
|   Long past infection | − | − | − | +‡ | + or − | +‡ |
| Chronic infection | | | | | | |
|   Chronic active hepatitis | +§ | + or − | + or − | +§ | + or − | −§ |
|   Chronic persistent hepatitis | +¶ | + or − | + or − | + | + or − | − |
|   Chronic HBV carrier state | +¶ | + or − | + or − | + | + or − | − |
| HBsAg immunization | − | − | − | − | − | + |

*HBsAg and HBeAg are occasionally undetectable in acute HBV infection.
†IgM anti-HBc may persist for over a year after acute infection when very sensitive assays are employed.
‡Total anti-HBc and anti-HBs may be detected together or separately long after acute infection.
§HBsAG-negative chronic active hepatitis may occur where total anti-HBc and anti-HBs may be detected together, separately, or not at all.
¶HBsAg-negative chronic persistent hepatitis and chronic HBV carriers have been observed.

**486–490. The answers are 486-b, 487-a, 488-e, 489-d, 490-c.**
*(Parslow, pp 219–227. Levinson, pp 63, 65, 103–107, 107–114, 313–321, 435–444, 461. Ryan, pp 243–249.)* Of the many methods available for antigen and antibody detection, LA, ELISA, RIA, CIE, and COA are the most widely used. Latex agglutination (LA) employs latex polystyrene particles sensitized by either antibody or antigen. LA is more sensitive than CIE and COA but slightly less sensitive than either RIA or EIA. LA has been used to detect *H. influenzae, Neisseria meningitidis,* and *S. pneumoniae* antigens in cerebrospinal fluid. LA has also been used for detection of cryptococcal antigen. Most recently, LA has been widely used for rapid detection of group A streptococcal antigen directly from the pharynx. The test is rapid (5 minutes), sensitive (approximately 90%), and specific (99%).

Coagglutination (COA), also an agglutination test, is slightly less sensitive than LA but is less susceptible to changes in environment (e.g., temperature). Most strains of coagulase-positive staphylococci have protein A in their cell wall. Protein A binds the Fc fragment of microbial antigens in body fluids. COA has also been used to rapidly type or group bacterial isolates.

Enzyme immunoassays (EIAs) can be either homogeneous (EMIT) or heterogeneous (ELISA). EMIT has been used primarily for assays of low-molecular-weight drugs. Its primary use in microbiology has been for assays of aminoglycoside antibiotics. EIAs vary as to the solid support used. A variety of supports can be used, such as polystyrene microdilution plates, paddles, plastic beads, and tubes. The number of layers in the antibody-antigen sandwich varies; usually as additional layers are added, detection sensitivity is increased. The two most common enzymes are horseradish peroxidase (HRP) and alkaline phosphatase (AP). β-Galactosidase has also been employed. Orthophenylene diamine is the most common substrate for HRP and p-nitrophenyl phosphate for AP. Because EIAs are usually read in the visible color range, the tests can be read qualitatively by eye or quantitatively by machine.

Counterimmunoelectrophoresis (CIE) was originally used for "Australia antigen" (HBsAg) but was soon replaced by RIA. For a decade, CIE was used to detect antigens in body fluids. CIE is not an easy technique. Its success depends on the control of many variables, including solid support, voltage, current, buffer, affinity and avidity of antibodies, charge on the antigen, and time of electrophoresing.

Radioimmunoassay involves the radiolabeling of either antibody or antigen (Ag) using $^{131}$Iodine ($^{131}$I) or $^{125}$I (radioisotopes). It measures very small quantities and can be used to detect hormones, carcinoembryonic antigen (CEA), hepatitis B Ag, steroids, prostaglandins, and morphine-related drugs in patient sera.

**491–495. The answers are 491-c, 492-a, 493-f, 494-e, 495-b.** (*Parslow, pp 221–224. Levinson, pp 344, 352–353, 437–438. Ryan, pp 245–247.*) The enzyme immunoassay (EIA, ELISA) has become a common method for the detection of either antibody or antigen in a patient specimen. The technique is based on building a "sandwich." For example, the following sandwich is made on what is called the *solid phase*. The solid phase is usually a plastic microtiter plate but can be a plastic paddle or even a nitrocellulose membrane. First, whole *Toxoplasma* organisms or purified antigenic components of *Toxoplasma* are added to the plate and the plate is washed off. Failure of one or more of the washing steps or inadequate washing usually causes high background color in the developed plate.

The *Toxoplasma* antigen-antibody complex must be detected by the addition of a second antibody to which is linked an enzyme such as horseradish peroxidase or alkaline phosphatase. The nature of this second antibody is dependent on whether one wishes to measure IgG or IgM. If the test is for IgG, then the second antibody is antihuman IgG conjugated to an enzyme. Following another wash cycle, the enzyme substrate is added to the plate and color develops in those wells where the sandwich is complete. If the patient's serum does not contain specific antibody, then the sandwich is not completed and there is no development of color. If the EIA is for detection of antigen, then the layers of the sandwich are as follows:

Specific antibody
Patient specimen (contain antigen)
Enzyme-labeled antibody specific for the antigen
Enzyme substrates

There are many variations of the test using a variety of antibodies, indicators such as fluorescence, and magnetic beads as solid phases. EIA is more sensitive than agglutination methods or complement fixation and slightly less sensitive than radioimmunoassay.

**496. The answer is d.** (*Parslow, pp 326–327, 739. Levinson, pp 429–430.*) GVHD occurs due to attack by the graft against the recipient. There are three requirements for GVHD rejection: (1) histocompatibility differences between the graft (donor) and host (recipient), (2) immunocompetent graft cells, and (3) immunodeficient host cell. Immunocompetent graft cells may be "passenger" lymphocytes or major cells transplanted, and must be present in the graft. Prevention of GVHD is essential, as there is no adequate treatment once it is established.

**497. The answer is c.** (*Parslow, pp 254–255. Levinson, pp 441–444.*) All blood for transfusion should be carefully matched to avoid transfusion reaction. As shown in the tables below, persons with group O blood have no A or B antigens on their erythrocytes and are thus considered to be universal donors. In contrast, persons with group AB blood have neither A nor B antibody and thus are universal recipients.

| | ABO BLOOD GROUPS | |
|---|---|---|
| **Group** | **Antigen on Red Cell** | **Antibody in Plasma** |
| A | A | Anti-B |
| B | B | Anti-A |
| AB | A and B | No anti-A or anti-B |
| O | No A or B | Anti-A and anti-B |

**COMPATIBILITY OF BLOOD TRANSFUSIONS BETWEEN ABO BLOOD GROUPS***

| | Recipient | | | |
|---|---|---|---|---|
| **Donor** | **O** | **A** | **B** | **AB** |
| O | Yes | Yes | Yes | Yes |
| A (AA or AO) | No | Yes | No | Yes |
| B (BB or BO) | No | No | Yes | Yes |
| AB | No | No | No | Yes |

*"Yes" indicates that a blood transfusion from a donor with that blood group to a recipient with that blood group is compatible, i.e., that no hemolysis will occur. "No" indicates that the transfusion is incompatible and that hemolysis of the donor's cells will occur.
*Reprinted, with permission, from Levinson W, Jawetz E.* Medical Microbiology and Immunology, *7e. New York: McGraw-Hill, 2002:412.*

**498–500. The answers are 498-b, 499-d, 500-h.** *(Parslow, pp 128–129, 401–405, 426–430. Levinson, pp 423–428. Levinson, pp 453–462. Harrison's, pp 1960–1967.)* Loss of tolerance by the immune system to certain self-components can lead to the formation of antibodies, causing tissue and organ damage. Such diseases are referred to as *autoimmune diseases*. There are a host of autoimmune diseases characterized by the autoantibodies. The presence of a "butterfly" rash is a classic cutaneous sign of SLE and is characterized by a rash over the bridge of the nose and on the cheeks.

# Bibliography

Bhushan V, et al. *First Aid for the USMLE Step 1: 2006.* New York: McGraw-Hill, 2006.

Brooks GF et al (ed). *Jawetz's Medical Microbiology,* 23/e. New York: McGraw-Hill, 2004.

Gilligan W et al (ed). *Cases in Medical Microbiology and Infectious Diseases,* 3/e. Washington, DC, ASM Press, 2003.

Kasper DL et al (eds). *Harrison's Principles of Internal Medicine,* 16/e. New York: McGraw-Hill, 2005.

Levinson W et al. *Medical Microbiology and Immunology,* 8/e. New York: McGraw-Hill, 2004.

Murray PR et al (ed). *Manual of Clinical Microbiology,* 8/e. Washington, DC: ASM Press, 2003.

Murray PR et al. *Medical Microbiology,* 5/e. St. Louis, MO: Mosby; 2005.

Parslow TG et al. *Medical Immunology,* 10/e. New York: McGraw-Hill, 2001.

Ryan KJ et al (ed). *Sherris Medical Microbiology,* 4/e. New York: McGraw-Hill, 2001.

# Index